D0453289

Department of Health

Report on Health and Social Subjects

45

Weaning and The Weaning Diet

Report of the Working Group on the Weaning Diet of the
Committee on Medical Aspects of Food Policy

London: HMSO

ISBN 0 11 321838 9

Preface

In 1991 the Committee on Medical Aspects of Food Policy (COMA) convened a Working Group to review nutritional aspects of the weaning of infants in the United Kingdom. The Working Group met on seven occasions, reviewed published information and invited expert reviews. It also received contributions following advertisement in the press. I am grateful to the Chairman and members of the Working Group and to all who gave freely of their time and knowledge.

Earlier reports from COMA have assessed how infants should best be fed in the first months after birth. By the time of weaning nutritional adequacy is potentially vulnerable. The stores of nutrients built up before birth are depleted and infants are dependent on a diet of mixed foods which they are sampling for the first time. When and why to wean and with which food, and how much should be given as the diet diversifies? What are the influences of family and society on how mothers feed their babies? These and other questions are discussed in this report which includes recommendations about how babies should be fed as well as the foods and drinks in their diets. Health problems related to the child's nutritional status have been examined, in particular there are recommendations about the management of iron deficiency anaemia including its prevention.

I welcome this report which I believe will lead the way to healthier weaning practices in the UK.

DR K C CALMAN
Chairman, Committee on Medical Aspects of Food Policy

Contents

Annexes

Committee on Medical Aspects of Food Policy
Working Group on Weaning and the Weaning Diet

Chairman

Professor F Cockburn	Department of Child Health, University of Glasgow.

Members

Dr I Hann	Department of Haematology, The Hospitals for Sick Children, London.
Mr R A Hendey	Infant and Dietetic Foods Association, London.
Dr R D Holt	Institute of Dental Surgery, Eastman Dental Hospital, London.
Dr J James	General Practitioner, Bristol.
Dr M Lawson	Institute of Child Health, London.
Dr I McKinlay	Royal Manchester Children's Hospital, Manchester.
Mrs P Margiotta	Bolton and Salford College of Midwifery and Nursing, Salford.
Dr E M E Poskitt	Department of Child Health, University of Liverpool and latterly, Dunn Nutrition Group, Keneba, The Gambia.
Dr A M Prentice	MRC Dunn Clinical Nutrition Centre, Cambridge.
Professor B A Wharton	The Old Rectory, Belbroughton, Worcs.

Observers

Dr B Fuge	Welsh Office, Cardiff.
Dr B Potter	Scottish Office Home and Health Department, Edinburgh.

Dr A Mairs	Department of Health and Social Services (Northern Ireland), Belfast.
Dr H A Tyler	Ministry of Agriculture, Fisheries and Food, London.
Dr J G Ablett	Department of Health, London.
Miss V Bahl	Department of Health, London.
Mr C Howard	Department of Health, London.
Mrs S Philogene	Department of Health, London.
Miss A F Robertson	Department of Health, London.
Dr H Walton	Department of Health, London.
Dr M J Wiseman	Department of Health, London.

Secretariat

Dr P C Clarke (Medical)	Department of Health, London.
Miss M J L Atkinson (Scientific)	Department of Health, London.
Miss A Halliday (Scientific)	Department of Health, London.
Mr R W Wenlock (Scientific)	Department of Health, London.
Mrs J Caro (Administrative)	Department of Health, London.
Mrs E Lohani (Administrative)	Department of Health, London.

Committee on Medical Aspects of Food Policy

Chairman

Dr KC Calman

Government Chief Medical Officer, Department of Health,

Members

Dr P J Aggett

Head of Nutrition, Diet and Health, Institute of Food Research, Norwich.

Professor KGMM Alberti

Professor of Medicine, University of Newcastle upon Tyne.

Dr S Bingham

MRC Dunn Clinical Nutrition Centre, Cambridge.

Dr J Chambers

Health Education Authority.

Professor F Cockburn

Department of Child Health, University of Glasgow.

Dr H Denner

Chief Scientist (Food), Ministry of Agriculture, Fisheries and Food, London.

Ms A Foster

Director, Scottish Consumer Council.

Dr G Fowler

Department of Public Health and Primary Care, Radcliffe Infirmary, Oxford.

Professor J Grimley Evans

Division of Geriatric Medicine, Nuffield Department of Clinical Medicine, University of Oxford.

Dr D Hine

Chief Medical Officer, Welsh Office.

Professor A Jackson

Professor of Human Nutrition, University of Southampton.

Professor W P T James

Director, Rowett Research Institute, Aberdeen.

Dr M Kemp

Medical Research Council, London.

Dr R E Kendall

Chief Medical Officer, The Scottish Office.

Dr J McKenna

Chief Medical Officer, Department of Health and Social Services, Northern Ireland.

Professor M Marmot

Department of Epidemiology and Public Health, UCL Medical School, University College, London.

Secretariat

Dr M Wiseman (Medical)

Department of Health, London.

Dr S Lader (Medical)

Department of Health, London.

Mr R Wenlock (Scientific)

Department of Health, London.

Mrs M Fry (Administrative)

Department of Health, London.

Dr S Martin (Administrative)

Department of Health, London.

Miss B Ferry (Administrative)

Department of Health, London.

Acknowledgements

The Working Group is grateful for the valuable assistance given as written contributions from the following organisations and experts.

Miss Jill Aitken	National Childbirth Trust, London.
Mr D W G Barrett	Wyeth Laboratories, Maidenhead.
Dr M Blair	Nottingham Health Authority, Nottingham.
British Dental Association	London.
British Paediatric Association	London.
Dr M B Duggan	Department of Paediatrics, University of Sheffield.
Dr D L J Freed	Department of Biological Sciences, University of Salford.
Dr P H Gordon	British Society of Paediatric Dentistry, Newcastle upon Tyne.
Dr P Hobson	Department of Oral Health and Development, University of Manchester.
Dr D Hodes	Department of Community Child Health, St Bartholomew's NHS Trust, London.
Dr R Hurrell	Nestle Research Centre, Vevey, Switzerland.
Ms E Keegan	SMA Nutrition, Maidenhead.
Ms J Kelham	East Dorset Health Authority, Community Health Services, Bournemouth.
Professor I Macdonald	Nutritional Consultative Panel of the Dairy Industry, Thames Ditton.
Dr I C MacKie	Department of Oral Health and Development, University of Manchester.
Maternity Alliance	London.

Dr P J Milla	Institute of Child Health, London.
Mrs A Morrant	Department of Dental Public Health, North Western Regional Health Authority, Manchester.
Ms S Murray	Newham Health Authority.
Miss A A Paul	MRC Dunn Nutrition Centre, Cambridge.
Dr J A Payne	Department of Child Life and Health, University of Edinburgh.
Professor M J Pippard	Department of Haematology, University of Dundee.
Dr A Prentice	MRC Dunn Nutrition Centre, Cambridge.
Dr G Roberts	Department of Orthodontics and Dentistry for Children, UMDS, Guy's Hospital Dental School.
Mr S S Stewart	Bounty Services Ltd, Borehamwood, Herts.
The Sugar Bureau	London.
Ms F Sutton	Newham Health Authority, London.
Professor J A Walker-Smith	Queen Elizabeth's Hospital for Sick Children, London.
Dr S A Williams	Department of Child Dental Health, University of Leeds.

1.   Recommendations

1.1   Recommendations for weaning practices

The process of weaning: Chapter 3

R1   The majority of infants should not be given solid foods before the age of four months, and a mixed diet should be offered by the age of six months.

R2   Infants should be supervised during meal times. Semi-solid food should be given from a spoon and not mixed with milk or other drink in a bottle. From six months of age, infants should be introduced to drinking from a cup and from age one year feeding from a bottle should be discouraged.

Food energy and macronutrients: Chapter 5

R3   The provision of adequate dietary energy to ensure normal growth and development should be a principal determinant of the diets of children under five years of age.

R4   An adequate intake of protein with a proper balance of essential amino acids should be ensured during weaning. A diet that is restricted, for whatever reason, should particularly offer a variety of foods at each meal providing a mixture of protein sources.

R5   Dietary recommendations from the COMA Working Group on Nutritional Aspects of Cardiovascular Disease concerning average levels of fat intakes do not apply before the age of two years, but apply in full from the age of five years. A flexible approach is recommended to the timing and extent of dietary change for individual children between the ages of two and five years.

R6   For groups of children the average intake of non-milk extrinsic sugars should be limited to about ten per cent of total dietary energy intake.

R7   Provided energy intake is adequate, the proportion of energy supplied as starch in the weaning diet should increase as the proportion derived from fat decreases.

Vitamins: Chapter 6

R8   Adequate vitamin status should be encouraged for mother and baby through a varied diet and moderate exposure to summer sunlight.

R9   Foods and drinks which provide good sources of vitamin C should be encouraged in the weaning diet.

1

R10   Breastfed infants under six months do not need vitamin supplementation provided the mother had an adequate vitamin status during pregnancy. From age six months, infants receiving breast milk as their main drink should be given supplements of vitamins A and D.

R11   Infants fed on manufactured milks do not need vitamin supplements provided their consumption of infant formula or follow on formula milk is more than 500 ml per day. If they are consuming infant formula or follow on milk in smaller amounts or they are being given cow's milk, vitamins A and D supplements should be given.

R12   Between the ages of one to five years, vitamins A and D supplements should be given unless adequate vitamin status can be assured from a diverse diet containing vitamins A and D rich foods and from moderate exposure to sunlight.

Minerals: Chapters 7 and 8

R13   Dietary sources of minerals should be provided by offering a variety of foods. Vitamin C in adequate amounts should be ensured with meals to assist absorption and this is particularly important if the diet is meat free. Continued use of iron-enriched infant formula or a follow on milk as a main drink after the first year should be considered if there are concerns about the adequacy of iron in the diet.

R14   There should be an adequate dietary intake of calcium. For young infants the dietary calcium to phosphorus ratio should be between 1.2 and 2.0 by weight (0.9:1 to 1.6:1 (molar)).

Milk and other drinks: Chapter 9

R15   Breast milk provides the best nourishment during the early months of life. Mothers should be encouraged and supported in breastfeeding for at least four months and may choose to continue to breastfeed as the weaning diet becomes increasingly varied.

R16   An infant who is not breastfed should receive infant formula or follow on milk. Follow on milk is not recommended as replacement for breast milk or infant formula before six months.

R17   Pasteurised whole cow's milk should only be used as a main milk drink after the age of one year. Intakes of iron and zinc and vitamins A and D should be ensured from other dietary sources or from supplements. Semi-skimmed cow's milk is not suitable as a drink before the age of two years but thereafter it may be introduced gradually if the child's energy and nutrient intake is otherwise adequate and if growth remains satisfactory. Fully skimmed cow's milk should not usually be introduced before the age of five years.

R18   Goat's and sheep's milks should not be given to infants, and if used after this age the milk must be pasteurised or boiled.

R19   Milk (also including breast milk, infant formula, follow on formula) or water should constitute the majority of the total drinks given. Other drinks should usually be confined to meal times and because of the risk to dental health, they should not be given in a feeding bottle or at bedtime.

Foods in the weaning diet: Chapter 10

R20   Non-wheat cereals, fruit, vegetables and potatoes are suitable first weaning foods. Salt should not be added and additional sugars should be limited to that needed for palatability of sour fruits. Between six and nine months of age the amount and variety of foods including meat, fish, eggs, all cereals and pulses should be increased and the number of "milk" feeds reduced. Food consistency should progress from pureed through minced/mashed to finely chopped. By the age of one year the diet should be mixed and varied.

R21   In the later states of weaning, three meals per day are suggested with two or three snacks in addition.

R22   The labels of commercial baby foods should provide consistent information which is understandable to parents.

R23   Foods given during weaning should be prepared, handled and stored in a hygienic way.

Food allergy: Chapter 11

R24   Where there is a family history of atopy or gluten enteropathy, mothers should be encouraged to breastfeed for six months or longer. Weaning before four months should particularly be discouraged and the introduction of foods traditionally regarded as allergenic should be delayed until six months at the earliest.

Vegetarian weaning and other dietary preferences: Chapter 11

R25   Infants being weaned on diets restricted in animal protein should particularly be offered a variety of foods at each meal. Protein sources should be mixed. Each meal should provide vitamin C, and an energy supplement from a fat source should be considered if there are doubts about the adequacy of energy intake.

R26   The range of commercial weaning foods should be enlarged to offer a wider choice to those with special cultural or religious dietary requirements and they should be appropriately labelled.

Growth and health: Chapter 12

R27   Infants and young children who are failing to thrive should be identified as early as possible, and a nutritional cause should be investigated.

Dental health: Chapter 13

R28   Weaning foods should usually be free of, or low in, non-milk extrinsic sugars including sugars derived from fruit juices and fruit concentrates. The range of commercial foods meeting these criteria should be increased. Foods and drinks which predispose to caries should be limited to main meal times. The sugars content of all weaning foods and drinks should be shown on food labels.

R29   Water supplies should be fluoridated to the optimum of one part per million. For infants and young children in areas that are not fluoridated, fluoride supplements may be advised where there is a particular risk of caries.

Educational and professional support: Chapter 14

R30   Professional staff who advise parents about weaning should be trained and should have access to dietetic expertise.

R31   Local nutrition policies for infants and children should be culturally acceptable to the communities concerned and should be developed through local multi-disciplinary cooperation including voluntary interests.

R32   All parents should receive nutrition education including information about weaning and the weaning diet. Education about feeding infants and young children should extend to the general public including school-children .

1.2   Recommendations for research

R33   Information about national patterns of diet and nutrition status should be available for the first two years of life.

R34   Research should be directed to understanding normal weaning and to establishing guidance on the rate at which the liquid diet of early infancy should change to a diet where solids provide the major part of energy and nutrient needs. The factors which predispose to disorders of weaning should be defined.

R35   The optimal quantities and qualities of dietary fats, during infancy and young childhood should be determined particularly through long-term studies.

R36   The effects on nutritional status of high intakes by young children of foods which are rich in non-starch polysaccharides and also often contain high phytate levels should be evaluated.

R37   Research should be encouraged on the biological functions of the anti-oxidant vitamins C and E and the carotenoids, their turnover, requirements in childhood and the possible benefits or detrimental effects of high intakes, also on the inter-relationship of these vitamins with fatty acids, selenium, iron, zinc, copper and manganese on the levels of antioxidant activity in developing infant tissues.

R38   The immediate and long-term effects of iron deficiency with and without anaemia during weaning on health and development should be defined more precisely.

R39   There should be further investigation of the relationship between iron status and the quality and quantity of dietary intakes of iron including the extent to which iron fortified milks and foods contribute absorbable iron.

R40   Means of preventing iron deficiency through effective nutrition education should be investigated further.

R41   Laboratory criteria for anaemia and for iron deficiency should be defined and used to determine the prevalence of anaemia and of iron deficiency in the general population of children under two years of age in the UK.

R42   There should be an assessment of the need for universal or population sub-group screening for iron deficiency anaemia in infants and young children and for the feasibility and acceptability of such a programme.

R43   The natural history of iron deficiency in infants and children in this country should be determined.

R44   The best method of intervention and follow up of populations of young children who have been screened for iron status should be determined.

R45   Research should be encouraged on calcium, phosphorus and magnesium metabolism in children. The interactions of these nutrients together with factors which modulate them, including diet and the mechanisms for adapting to diets poor in these nutrients should be clarified.

R46   Investigations should be encouraged to determine the optimal balance of iron, zinc and copper in the weaning diet.

R47   There should be further investigation of dietary factors which initiate atopic disorders.

R48   There should be further research into the nutritional causes of failure to thrive.

R49   Criteria for defining fatness in young children should be standardised. The determinants of fatness in young children, its prevalence and population changes in degrees of fatness should be examined and short and long-term consequences assessed.

R50   Priority should be given to continuing investigations into the effect of diet and nutrition of the infant and young child on health in childhood and adult life.

R51   Methods should be developed to foster professional and public awareness of the importance of the weaning diet to dental health and to promote good practices especially in groups at risk of dental disease.

R52   More effective strategies for public education should be developed and they should be based on information from research.

2. Introduction

2.1 **Background** Nutrition in the early years of life is a major determinant of growth and development and it also influences adult health (para 12.3). The first report from the Committee on Medical Aspects of Food Policy (COMA) on Present Day Practice in Infant Feeding in 1974[1], was followed by two further reviews[2,3]. These reports focused on nutrition in infancy with comment about good nutrition in the pre-school years. This present report addresses the growing interest in the infant and young child during weaning, in the change from milk to a fully mixed diet, and in nutritional status during weaning. Recently COMA recommended that there should be less total fat and saturated fatty acids in the diets of adults[4], and questions have arisen about whether this should also be applied to the composition of the diet during weaning and early childhood. COMA convened a Working Group on Weaning and the Weaning Diet in 1991.

2.2 Terms of reference of the Working Group

2.2.1 The terms of reference of the working group were "To review the nutrition of young children during weaning and to make recommendations".

2.2.2 The Working Group considered the nutrition of infants and young children between the ages of about 6 weeks to about 2 years. Although the introduction of solid foods as early as 6 weeks is not recommended, it is known to occur (see Annex 1). The upper age limit was more difficult to agree because it was recognised that first solids are followed by a period which varies from child to child when the diet may be highly individual before the pattern of the school years becomes established. This report focuses on the first 2 years of life as being the likely limits of the weaning period, but acknowledges the continuing importance of diet and nutrition for older children.

2.2.3 The definition of weaning adopted by the Working Group was the process of expanding the diet to include foods and drinks other than breast milk or infant formula. Weaning allows the infant to meet changing nutritional needs and to become less nutritionally dependent on milk.

2.3 The weaning diet in this country

2.3.1 Studying the diets of young children is not straightforward. Qualitative data give a general picture of what foods are being offered to children at this age but precise conclusions about what constitutes a customary diet during weaning are difficult because of frequent changes in diet as the child gets older, and the different rates at which children mature. Gathering quantitative intake data presents an even greater challenge especially when food remains uneaten or is spat out. Nevertheless, because of the importance of this period in a child's development, several studies have been attempted over the last 25 years. There are three important sources of national data: a large and detailed survey in 1967 of children aged 6 months to 4½ years[5], four cross sectional surveys at 5 yearly intervals of infant feeding practices[6,7,8,9], and a dietary survey in 1986 of infants aged 6 to 12 months[10]. This last survey, commissioned by the Ministry of Agriculture, Fisheries and Food (MAFF), has been drawn on extensively in preparing this report. A brief description of these surveys and other local surveys and some of the more significant results are at Annex 1.

2.3.2   The Departments of Health and the Ministry of Agriculture, Fisheries and Food jointly sponsor the National Diet and Nutrition Survey programme. Individuals from defined population groups are selected so that, as a group, they provide a representative sample of the whole population. The groups are age related. Following the completion of the survey of adults aged 18 to 64 years, the population of pre-school children aged 1½ to 4½ years has been the most recently surveyed group. Twelve months fieldwork was completed in June 1993 and a report is in preparation[11]. Preliminary results from the survey of pre-school children have been used to a limited extent in this COMA report.

2.3.3   The survey of pre-school children was preceded by a feasibility study to validate methodology[12]. Apart from collecting questionnaire and dietary data, this study included an assessment of energy expenditure using doubly labelled water. These data have been used in this report.

2.3.4   These sources of data vary in the ages of the subjects and in how long ago the surveys were done. Up to date information should be available about diet and nutrition in the UK during the first two years of life.

The Working Group recommends that

●   **information about national patterns of diet and nutrition status should be available for the first two years of life (para 2.3.4).**

2.4   **Meetings of the Working Group**   The Working Group held seven meetings, one was held jointly with the COMA Panel on Child Nutrition. Submissions of evidence were invited. The Working Group is grateful to those who submitted evidence whose names are listed earlier.

2.5   **Definitions and abbreviations**

2.5.1   An *infant* is a child who has not attained the age of one year.
A *young child* is a child aged from one to three years.
Weaning is the process of expanding the diet to include foods and drinks other than breast milk or infant formula.

2.5.2   mmol millimol (equivalent to atomic/molecular weight in mg)
g   gram

kg   kilogram (1000 g)

mg   milligram (one-thousandth of 1 g)

µg   microgram (one-millionth of 1 g)

ng   nanogram (one-thousand-millionth of 1 g)

l   litre

ml   millilitre (one-thousandth of 1 litre).

kJ   kiloJoule (1000 Joules). A unit used to measure the energy value of food (1 kJ = 0.239 kcal).

MJ   megaJoule (one million Joules).

kcal   kilocalories (1000 calories). A unit used to measure the energy value of food (1 kcal = 4.18 kJ).j16

d   day

3. The process of weaning

The Working Group recommends that

● the majority of infants should not be given solid foods before the age of four months, and a mixed diet should be offered by the age of six months (para 3.1.2);

● infants should be supervised during meal times. Semi-solid foods should be given from a spoon and not mixed with milk or other drink in a bottle. From six months of age, infants should be introduced to drinking from a cup and from age one year feeding from a bottle should be discouraged (para 3.6.1);

● research should be directed to understanding normal weaning and to establishing guidance on the rate at which the liquid diet of early infancy should change to a diet where solids provide the major part of energy and nutrient needs. The factors which predispose to disorders of weaning should be defined (para 3.1.1).

3.1 Introduction

3.1.1 Weaning enables infants to meet their changing nutritional needs as they become less dependent on milk. It coincides with a period of rapid growth and development when an adequate diet is crucial to meet nutrient needs. The Working Group found only limited information on which to base recommendations for best weaning practices. Most of the body's systems are maturing and growing rapidly at this age and the rate of weaning should take account of considerable individual variation. Weaning should not proceed at a rate which, because it is too slow or too fast, leaves the diet nutritionally deficient or the gut mucosa damaged. Weaning too early or too late, or with inappropriate foods, or in an inappropriate manner, can result in behavioural and health problems and in family stress. The weaning process should be investigated further to help to define practical recommendations.

3.2 When should weaning begin?

3.2.1 There are health benefits for infants who are exclusively breastfed during the first months of life (para 9.1). The Working Group recommends that solid foods should be introduced between the ages of 4 to 6 months. By this age the infant's physiology and development have matured to cope with the weaning diet and most infants are ready to experience new tastes and textures. Infants should be consuming solids when a more energy and nutrient dense diet is needed than can be provided by milk alone. On the other hand, weaning should not start before neuromuscular coordination has developed sufficiently to allow the infant to eat solids, nor before the gut and kidney have matured to cope with a more diverse diet. The first report from COMA about infant feeding made a similar recommendation about the age at which weaning should begin[1]. The second and third reports on Present Day Practice in Infant Feeding stressed the wide range of rates of growth and of maturing in the months after birth and acknowledged that some infants might begin weaning at 3 months[2,3]. While the individual needs of infants may occasionally lead to starting a mixed diet at 3 months, the Working Group on Weaning and the Weaning Diet recommends that a start to weaning no earlier than age 4 months is the most appropriate advice for the great majority of infants.

3.2.2 *Increasing energy and nutrient needs* Infants double their birth weight in the first 4 to 5 months of life and eventually their dietary needs can no longer be met by fluids. The absorption of nutrients from breast milk is highly efficient and, provided the infant consumes good amounts and the mother is well nourished, no other foods begin to be needed until about 4 months of age. Solids, given with breast milk, can reduce the absorption of nutrients in the milk (para 7.3), and there may be advantage if a diverse diet is introduced only when the infant is ready to eat solids in amounts large enough to compensate for any associated reduction in the bioavailability of nutrients. By 6 months, if the infant is still unweaned the amounts of energy, protein and vitamins A and D (para 6.6) are particularly likely to be inadequate. Additional sources of absorbable iron and zinc are needed from the diet at generally no later than the age of 6 months if the child is not to become iron deficient and at risk of anaemia (para 7.3). Similar guidelines about when to begin weaning apply to bottle fed infants although the intake of several nutrients and their bioavailability from infant formula are significantly different from breast milk.

3.2.3 *Development of neuromuscular coordination* The neuromuscular co-ordination needed to eat solid foods develops during the early months of post natal life. Young infants have poor head control and, before about 3 months old, head and back support is so weak that it is difficult to hold infants in a position where they can be fed and can easily swallow semi-solid foods. By 4 months, most infants can maintain posture if supported sitting in a chair. The newborn sucks at food and tends to spit out food placed on the anterior part of the tongue. Before 3 months infants cannot easily form a bolus to move solid food from the front to the back of the mouth but infants of 5 months should be able to take soft pureed foods from a spoon, form a bolus and swallow it. Infants of 5 months hold objects and put them to their mouths or may pick them up to suck. These skills can be encouraged by providing foods for the infant to hold. Infants can chew from about 6 months old. If not encouraged, this ability may not develop readily and teaching older infants to chew can be difficult[13]. From about 7 months, infants learn to shut their mouths, turn their heads and indicate refusal to feed. This can be used manipulatively and may make weaning particularly difficult if the child has not yet accepted new tastes and textures (para 12.2).

3.2.4 *Maturation of the infant kidney* A newborn baby has limited renal capacity to conserve fluids and to excrete a solute load (para 8.4). Breast milk or infant formula are low solute, high volume foods and appropriate at this early age. By 4 months renal function has matured considerably and infants

11

can conserve water better and can deal with varying solute concentrations. Older infants can cope with a weaning diet which gradually reduces the volume of fluid intake while increasing the concentration of nutrients.

3.2.5 *Development of the gastro-intestinal tract* The secretion of gastric, intestinal and pancreatic enzymes is not fully developed in the young infant[14]. For infants being breastfed, breast milk contains enzymes which contribute to the hydrolysis of food in the gut lumen. Enzymes from the salivary glands are relatively important in the early months and salivary amylase begins to break down complex polysaccharides in the mouth and stomach while lingual lipase begins the digestion of fats. The brush border of the jejunum secretes digestive enzymes and allows the absorption of nutrients on specific transporter proteins. By 3 months of age increased gastric acid secretion assists gastric pepsin to digest protein. At 9 months trypsin and lipase are produced by the pancreas at rates similar to those in older children. Pancreatic amylase begins to make an effective contribution to digestion between the ages of 12 and 18 months. Water and electrolytes are absorbed in both the small and large intestines. The absorption of all nutrients becomes more efficient with age and the growing intestine offers an increased number of transporter sites for nutrients to be absorbed[15].

3.2.6 Gut motility depends on the integrity of the enteric nerves and smooth muscle layers of the intestine. The pattern of gut motility is determined by neurochemical coding of the neurones of the enteric nervous system. In the fasting state, contractile activity is cyclical and associated with surges in secretion of the polypeptide hormones motilin and somatostatin. When the infant eats, this activity becomes continuous. Eating and foods influence the release of cholecystokinin, gastrin, neurotensin and pancreatic polypeptide which all stimulate gut motility. Fat is most potent at stimulating gut motility, protein somewhat less and glucose initiates very little[16].

3.2.7 *Age of first giving solids in Britain* The proportions of infants who had been given solid foods by 8 weeks, 3 months and 4 months are shown in Table 3.1. In 1990, 9 per cent of mothers in Britain had given their babies solid food by 6 weeks, and by 8 weeks one in five babies had started to be weaned. Bottle feeding was associated with early introduction of solids. Early weaning was more likely in the North of England and Scotland, if the mothers were smokers and more likely in social class V than in social classes I and II[9]. In a survey commissioned by the Ministry of Agriculture, Fisheries and Food of infants aged 6 to 12 months[10], mothers were asked to recall the age at which they first gave foods other than milk. Sixteen per cent said they had given solids to their infants by 8 weeks of age and by 3 months just over half of the infants were being given solids.

3.2.8 The ages at which solids are reported first to have been introduced may not give a picture of the infant's diet as a whole. Some young babies receive new foods in no more than "taster" amounts and rely on milk as their main food for a long time. Others receive rapidly increasing proportions of solids in the diet. It is commonly observed that foods are added to a bottle of infant formula, for instance crumbled rusk, or baby rice, which is not always acknowledged as "introducing solids". Mothers may not report this practice, especially as many are aware that it is not advised by professionals. Because of the diversity of when and how solid foods are first introduced into the diets of young infants, guidance about good practice must recognise and build on current practices if improvements are to be encouraged.

Table 3.1 *Proportions of infants who have been given solids at different ages - UK studies (see Annex I)*

Study population Year of study	Proportion of infants given solids Age of infant		
	8 weeks	3 months	4 months
Nationally representative samples of infants			
1975: E.W[6].	49%	85%	97%
1980: E.W.S[7].	24%	56%	89%
1985: E.W.S[8].	24%	62%	90%
1990: UK[9].	19%	68%	94%
National study			
1986: E.W.S[10].	16%	52%	84%

E: England, W: Wales, S: Scotland, UK: United Kingdom

3.3 Antigens and the infant gut

3.3.1 Antigens can either be excluded or dealt with once they have been absorbed. As the gut matures in the early months of infancy, the permeability of the gut wall to large molecules decreases, a change which has been called "closure"[17]. By 3 to 4 months post-term only molecules less than 4 angstrom can pass through the intestinal wall. Immunoglobin A which is secreted by the small intestine influences the absorption of macromolecules and the formation of antibodies.

3.3.2 Foods which have commonly been associated with an adverse antigenic response include cow's milk, soya protein, gluten, egg, fish and chicken as well as rice (which is not often recognised as allergenic) (para 11.1). A recent study from Scotland found that persistent cough was more common in infants who had been given solid foods before 12 weeks than in those who were introduced to solids at an older age, although the study could not determine whether this was a manifestation of recurrent respiratory infection or of atopic disease[18]. Infants and young children occasionally present with intractable diarrhoea which is difficult to manage. Eighty per cent of such cases are due to enteropathic disorders of which 60 to 70 per cent are caused by food sensitivity which responds favourably to a diet which excludes the allergen[19]. In the past 20 years the incidence of gluten intolerance as a cause of protracted diarrhoea has dropped substantially and the age of onset of coeliac disease has increased[20]. This change has been ascribed to the adoption of recommendations against introducing solids at very young ages.

3.4 Taste and the acquisition of food habits

3.4.1 Taste influences food acceptance and preferences at all ages. The newborn modify their patterns of sucking in response to altered tastes. Taste responses appear similar to those of older children although there is considerable individual variation. Very young infants appear to gain pleasure from consuming moderate concentrations of sucrose solution but they are less eager to accept strong concentrations[21]. There is conflicting evidence about the response to salt. In a comparative study, young infants did not appear to discriminate between two infant formulae identical apart from different concentrations of sodium chloride[22]. On the other hand concentrated sodium chloride solutions dropped in the mouth evoked salivation and rejection[23]. Sour and bitter tastes are generally associated with negative responses from the newborn[21].

3.4.2 Weaning depends on the infant learning to enjoy new foods. Foods, which are initially rejected, are often readily accepted after repeated experiences. A recent study of 36 infants found that those who had been breastfed increased the quantity of pureed peas and beans consumed at weaning more rapidly than did the infants who had previously been fed infant formula exclusively[24]. The cause suggested for this difference may have been the habituation of the breastfed infant to a range of flavours and odours transmitted in the mother's milk. This suggests that breastfeeding may facilitate the acceptance of solid foods.

3.4.3 Foods are chosen because of sensory stimuli of taste, texture, smell and the appearances of colour, shape and presentation. In the 1920s, 15 infants with no experience of solid foods were allowed to self-select their diets until they were 6 years old. Their choices provided an increasingly diverse diet which was nutritionally adequate for health, growth and development[25]. Although this experiment might suggest that the infants were innately capable of selecting a satisfactory diet, in more normal circumstances diverse environmental factors also influence food preferences[26]. Parents want their children to learn to eat a healthy diet, and much of the advice about weaning practices is directed at this goal. Society and family exert pressures to conform to traditions, cultures and beliefs, and as they grow up young people absorb attitudes to buying, preparing, cooking and serving food. Individual circumstances, such as food allergies or personal convictions, also influence the development of food habits. For young adults there are other determinants of patterns of eating according to employment, economic status and social pressures. Boys, girls, young men, and young women are all likely as groups to have different eating patterns. All of these factors contribute to the parents' own attitudes to eating which help to determine how they chose a weaning diet for their child. A major research programme has been commissioned by the Economic and Social Research Council. It will examine the range of social influences on food choice. One of the research modules on the psychological determinants of children's food preferences is due to be completed in 1995.

3.4.4 The extent to which early acquired eating patterns influence dietary choices in adolescence and adult life is unknown. High rates of preference for sweet tastes among 2 year olds has been related to the regular consumption of sugar water whereas infants who had not been given sugar solutions had no strong preference for "sweet tasting foods"[21]. The relationship between early intake and later preference for sodium chloride is not known, although most under-fives show an increasing liking for salty foods as they grow older. It is unknown whether the perception of taste remains the same throughout childhood or whether it is modified by maturation of the sensory receptors. Commonsense suggests that healthy patterns of family eating do influence a child to choose to eat likewise and that these habits tend to persist.

3.5 Teething

3.5.1 The eruption of teeth contributes to the development of biting and chewing and increases the child's ability to explore different food textures. Teething begins, on average, at 6 months when weaning is in progress. It may be accompanied by discomfort, irritability, cheek flushing and drooling but it does not cause marked constitutional upset. Some infants find relief from discomfort by biting on a hard object such as a solid teething ring. Teeth are not essential for good nutrition at this stage and the presence or absence of teeth need not exert any great influence on how and when an individual infant is weaned although the foods and drinks should not predispose to dental decay. Caries can begin as soon as teeth erupt. Weaning practices can have a major influence on both immediate and future dental health (para 13.2).

3.6 Practical recommendations for weaning

3.6.1 Weaning foods smell, taste and feel different from breast or formula milks, they are offered in mouthfuls while milk and other drinks come in a continuous stream. Successful weaning has to overcome the aversion to new eating experiences which is common to most infants. Behaviour during weaning can be exasperating with refusal of food, spitting it out, sicking it up, tipping it over, dipping hands in it, squeezing and smearing it, wanting more, demanding something else, or a faster or slower supply. Infants quickly learn to try to get their own way and may reject savoury food if they know that eventually a dessert, which they prefer, will be given. Much of this behaviour, which is common, is normal and an expression of individuality on the part of the child. Infants need foods and eating implements with which to experiment and time and encouragement to learn. They adapt more successfully to the dietary changes of weaning if solid foods are offered from a spoon or are given as finger foods for the infant to hold and experiment. As sipping and swallowing replace sucking, feeding from a cup should begin (modified cups with lids are useful to avoid spills in the early stages). Bottle feeding should be discouraged after the age of 12 months. Solids should not be crumbled into drinks or given in bottles. This practice delays learning the food handling skills needed to diversify the diet. Furthermore, bottle feeding sweetened solids carries a risk of dental caries (para 13.2).

3.6.2 Dummy sucking is common in this country. There is no information about whether this habit is associated with particular patterns of sucking, chewing or accepting new foods. Dummies promote the swallowing of air. They are frequently infected with Candida albicans and a proportion of dummy suckers have oral thrush which may resist treatment until the dummy is discarded[27].

3.6.3 Infants should be supervised and encouraged during meal times. Some parents believe that their infant will learn good eating habits by being integrated into family meals, others feed their infants separately at a quiet time when the baby can receive undivided attention and can concentrate on the learning experience. Both approaches can be fully satisfactory. Parents and babies make individual contributions to family relationships. Health professionals and other advisors need to be sensitive to these family dynamics and support parents' confidence in their ability to wean their baby successfully (para 14.1).

4. Dietary Reference Values

4.1 Dietary Reference Values (DRVs) for energy and nutrients were most recently set for the UK in 1991[28]*. DRVs define the range of dietary requirements in different groups of individuals. They take account of the biological variation between individuals which determines differing energy and nutrient needs. Normal metabolic needs for healthy individuals, such as the needs for growth, are taken into account, although the DRVs make no allowances for the different energy and nutrient needs imposed by diseases. DRVs are used to assist in interpreting dietary intake information. They provide yardsticks for dietary guidance and planning and are used for food labelling purposes.

4.2 For most nutrients the DRVs comprise three levels of intake: the Estimated Average Requirement of a group for that nutrient (EAR); the intake sufficient to cover the needs of those in the group with the highest requirements (Reference Nutrient Intake – RNI); and the intake sufficient only for those with lowest requirements (Lower Reference Nutrient Intake – LRNI). For energy, and for fat and carbohydrate, whose main nutritional purpose is the provision of energy, it is important to consume neither insufficient nor excess and only an Estimated Average Requirement is given. Where there were insufficient data to set DRVs but the function of the nutrient (pantothenic acid, biotin, vitamin E, vitamin K, manganese, molybdenum, chromium and fluoride) is important, values for an intake, or range of intakes, were derived to meet the need of all individuals. This was called a "safe intake", at which level there was judged to be minimal risk of undesirable effects from too low or high an intake in any individual.

(i) *Estimated Average Requirement* (EAR) – The estimate of the average dietary requirement for food energy or a nutrient.

(ii) *Reference Nutrient Intake* (RNI) – The amount of a nutrient that is enough for almost every individual, even someone who has high needs for the nutrient in the distribution of individual requirements. It represents a value two notional standard deviations above the EAR. The level of intake is, therefore, considerably higher than most people need and individuals consuming the RNI are most unlikely to be deficient. If the average intake of a group is at the level of the RNI, then the risk of deficiency in the group is very low.

(iii) *Lower Reference Nutrient Intake* (LRNI) – A nutrient intake level

---

* This publication was reprinted with textual corrections in 1994; at the same time, in the section on fluoride, the safe intake levels were amended[29].

17

representing two notional standard deviations below the EAR. This amount is enough for only the small number of people who have the lowest needs. People habitually eating less than the LRNI will almost certainly be deficient.

4.3 Data about the nutrient needs of children is limited. For several nutrients, DRVs were set by extrapolating between the values for young adults and those for infants based on the composition of breast milk. Thus, between the ages of 6 and 24 months most of the DRVs provide a small increase with age. It is important to recognise that these values are based on sparse experimental data and, while providing serviceable best estimates, should not be interpreted as well founded statements of need. DRVs vary with age, sex and weight. Because the weights of boys and girls are significantly different only from 11 years and over, the same DRVs for nutrients were set for both sexes under 11 years. The following reference weights for population groups were adopted.

Age (months)	Weight (kg)
0-3 (formula fed only)*	5.9
4-6	7.7
7-9	8.9
10-12	9.8
12-36	12.6

* The DRVs for infants aged 0-3 months were set only for those being fed with infant formula. COMA saw no value in setting DRVs for breast fed babies of this age.

The DRVs for individual nutrients are considered in the context of the relevant chapters.

5. Food energy and macronutrients during weaning

5.1 Energy

The Working Group recommends that

● **the provision of adequate dietary energy to ensure normal growth and development should be a principle determinant of the diets of children under five years of age (para 5.1.5).**

5.1.1 The Estimated Average Requirements (EARs) for energy for children to 2 years of age are given below. The EARs for boys and girls were assumed to be identical when expressed on a body weight basis, so, because they are heavier, boys have greater EARs for energy than girls of the same age[28] (Table 5.1).

Table 5.1 *Estimated Average Requirements (EARs) of energy for children aged 0-24 months*

Age months	Energy intake per kg bodyweight kJ(kcal)/kg/d	EAR kJ(kcal)/d	
		Boys*	Girls*
1	480 (115)	1990 (480)	1920 (460)
3	420 (100)	2570 (610)	2390 (570)
6	400 (95)	3200 (760)	2980 (710)
9	400 (95)	3680 (880)	3420 (820)
12	400 (95)	4020 (960)	3800 (910)
18	400 (95)	4520 (1080)	3800 (910)
24	400 (95)	4960 (1190)	4720 (1130)

* Calculated using standard body weights for boys and girls described in para 4.3

5.1.2 The EARs for energy are lower than earlier UK estimates[30]. An expert WHO/FAO/UNU consultation in 1985 recommended an increase in energy requirement towards the end of the first year of life but this was based solely on food energy *intake* records[31]. Recent UK data do not support the need for this. Current assessments of energy requirements are now also able to draw on the results of doubly labelled water techniques of measurement which reflect the total energy *expenditure* in free living infants and children. The results suggest that earlier recommendations for energy were too high[32]. Modern surveys of the dietary energy intakes of infants also show significantly lower

19

mean levels than had been recorded previously[33]. Slightly slower mean growth rates and reduced degrees of adiposity have been observed at the same time as the mean energy intake fall[33]. The significance of these observations for the health of the infant remains unclear. A proportion of energy is needed for growth, but after the first 6 months of life this accounts for less than 3 per cent of the total dietary energy requirement[32].

5.1.3 The metabolisable energy intake from food is calculated from conversion factors developed by Southgate and Durnin[34]. These factors are likely to be inappropriate to assess energy intakes in young infants because of the inefficiency of fat absorption compared with that in adults, although probably satisfactory for older infants. Further uncertainties arise about food intake records in this age group because of the considerable variations in energy intakes between individuals of the same age and from day to day in the same child[35].

5.1.4 The dietary energy intakes of infants from 6 months recorded in the 1986 MAFF survey[10] are shown in Table 5.2 with the EARs for 7 to 9 months and for 10 to 12 months of age. The mean energy intakes of all groups slightly exceeded the respective EAR values; the median values for girls were lower than the mean values and closer to the EARs.

Table 5.2 *Recorded daily energy intakes of British infants[10] compared with daily Estimated Average Requirements (EAR) (kJ (kcal))[28]*

	Mean	Median	EAR
Males 6-8 months	3520 (836)	3520 (837)	3440 (825)*
Females 6-8 months	3340 (795)	3170 (751)	3200 (765)*
Males 9-12 months	4040 (960)	4000 (950)	3850 (920)**
Females 9-12 months	3810 (905)	3540 (841)	3610 (865)**

*   EAR for 7-9 months of age
** EAR for 10-12 months of age

5.1.5 During the first six months of life growth rate is greater than at any time during post-natal life. In older infancy, although the growth rate declines, it remains high compared with childhood. It is therefore most important that adequate food energy is assured throughout weaning. Fat contributes 50 per cent of the energy in breast milk and in infant formula and is the main source of energy for infants less than 6 months old. Proportionate contributions of fat, carbohydrate and protein to the dietary energy intakes of infants aged 6 to 12 months in the MAFF national survey are shown in Figure 5.1. Although carbohydrate provided the major contribution to dietary energy, the contribution from fat continued to be important. As the infant's diet diversifies, energy rich foods should continue to be included, and in particular, the diet should not be modified specifically to lower fat content by the inclusion of low fat foods before the age of 2 years (para 5.3). Diets which are energy deficient lead to slower growth and failure to thrive (para 12.1).

20

Table 5.1 The contributions of carbohydrate, protein and fat to the mean dietary energy intakes of British infants aged 6-12 months (MAFF)[10]

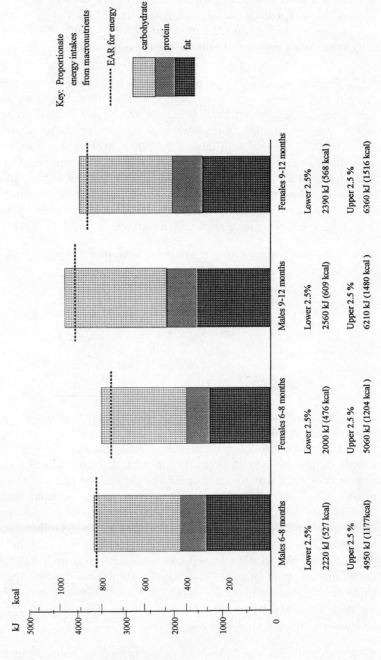

Key: Proportionate energy intakes from macronutrients

- - - EAR for energy

carbohydrate
protein
fat

Males 6-8 months
Lower 2.5 %
2220 kJ (527 kcal)
Upper 2.5 %
4950 kJ (1177 kcal)

Females 6-8 months
Lower 2.5 %
2000 kJ (476 kcal)
Upper 2.5 %
5060 kJ (1204 kcal)

Males 9-12 months
Lower 2.5 %
2560 kJ (609 kcal)
Upper 2.5 %
6210 kJ (1480 kcal)

Females 9-12 months
Lower 2.5 %
2390 kJ (568 kcal)
Upper 2.5 %
6360 kJ (1516 kcal)

kJ   kcal
5000
4000   1000
3000   800
        600
2000
        400
1000
        200
0

daily dietary energy intake

5.2 Protein

The Working Group recommends that

- **an adequate intake of protein with a proper balance of essential amino acids should be ensured during weaning. A diet that is restricted, for whatever reason, should particularly offer a variety of foods at each meal providing a mixture of protein sources (para 5.2.2).**

5.2.2 Protein intake is a crucial determinant of linear growth. The RNI for protein for infants aged 0 to 3 months is calculated from the COMA recommendations for artificial feeds for the young infant[36]. The RNIs for infants aged 4 months and older and for young children are based on WHO/FAO/UNU values[31] (Table 5.2). When expressed per kg body weight, daily dietary requirements decline from 1.4 g/kg at 4 months to 0.9 g/kg in the second year of life[31]. These figures assume complete digestibility of the protein and are based on values for total nitrogen in human milk without adjustments for the 20 per cent which is non-protein nitrogen in the form of urea, creatinine, uric acid, amino acids and nucleotides[37].

Table 5.3 *Reference Nutrient Intakes for protein for children aged 0-24 months*[31,28]

Age months	RNI g/d
0 - 3	12.5
4 - 6	12.7
7 - 9	13.7
10 - 12	14.9
13 - 24	14.5

5.2.3 Infants in the UK, whose diets rapidly diversify and who by the age of 9 months are regularly consuming meat, fish, eggs or reasonably quantities of milk, are unlikely to be protein deficient. There may be difficulties where infants do not eat animal products (para 11.2). Most plant foods are low in protein compared with foods of animal origin and the proteins from any single plant, unlike animal proteins, do not contain all the essential amino acids. If plant protein sources are mixed the full range of essential amino acids is more likely to be met[38,39]. The presence of non-starch polysaccharides (para 5.6) may reduce the bioavailability of amino acids. Adding 4g of "fibre" to the diets of 9 year old South African children increased their daily nitrogen and fat excretion by over a third[40]. Enzyme inhibitors active against lipase, chymotrypsin, and trypsin are common particularly in legumes[41] and some legumes also have tryptic like enzyme activity. The adverse effects of both enzymic activity and inhibitors may be reduced by cooking.

5.2.4 Soya protein based infant formulae meet the requirements for essential amino acids for young infants. They continue to provide a useful protein source for children beyond the first year of life. The essential amino acid content and the quantity of protein in soya infant formulae are important adjuncts to vegetarian weaning diets[42] (para 9.6).

5.3   Fat

The Working Group recommends that

● **dietary recommendations from the COMA Working Group on Nutritional Aspects of Cardiovascular Disease concerning average levels of fat intakes do not apply before the age of two years, but apply in full from the age of five years. A flexible approach is recommended to the timing and extent of dietary change for individual children between the ages of two and five years (para 5.3.4).**

● **the optimal quantities and qualities of dietary fats, during infancy and young childhood should be determined particularly through long-term studies (para 5.3.9).**

5.3.1   Fat is the major contributor to the total energy intake of infants in the first months of life, but by 6 months fat contributes proportionately less than carbohydrate (Figure 5.1). The high energy density of fat allows infants and young children to obtain their energy requirements from a manageable volume of food. Over 50 per cent of the energy in breast milk comes from fat[43] and the same is true for whole cow's milk[44]. By law infant formula and follow-on formula must provide 30 to 56.6 per cent of energy from fat[45].

5.3.2   Data from six dietary surveys of British children under 3 years of age[5,46,47,33,48,10,12] were analysed to provide the mean percentages of dietary energy derived from fat for each group studied (Figure 5.2). The infants under 4 months were breastfed, and, predictably the proportion of energy from fat was about 50 per cent. The percentage of energy derived from fat fell with the onset of weaning. From about age 8 months to 3 years the proportion of dietary energy from fat was between 35 to 40 per cent or less. A similar pattern was observed in Holland. About 100 Dutch children randomly selected as representative for each year of age between 1 and 5 years had average percentages of energy from fat of 31.7 per cent at 1 year, 34.0 per cent at 2 years, 36.1 per cent at 3 years, 36.2 per cent at 4 years and 36.4 per cent at 5 years[49]. These observations suggest that, as the high fat diet of breast or formula milk is replaced by weaning foods, the contribution from fat to the energy intake falls rapidly before rising to between 35 to 40 per cent by the age of 2 years. Good data on the percentage of energy from fat in a representative sample of British children aged 1½ to 4½ years are expected by autumn 1994 from the National Diet and Nutrition Survey (para 2.3).

5.3.3   Figure 5.3 compares the proportions of energy from fat in the weaning diets of children from communities originating from the North Indian subcontinent living in Sheffield[50] (Annex I) with those of British children who were predominantly white (values are the same as those shown in Figure 5.2). Fat tended to provide a higher proportion of energy in the diets of Asian children at all ages from 6 to 30 months and this was ascribed to high intakes of infant formula and cow's milk. Differences, such as these, in weaning practices between communities need to be taken into account when offering dietary guidance or nutrition education (para 11.2; para 14.3).

Figure 5.2   Proportions of food energy from fat

British infants and young children, 6 studies, 1967-90

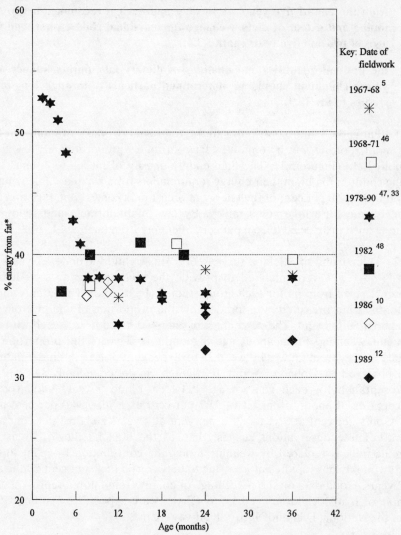

Key: Date of fieldwork

1967-68 [5]

1968-71 [46]

1978-90 [47, 33]

1982 [48]

1986 [10]

1989 [12]

*Two values at the same age from one study, provides results for boys and girls separately,
(% energy from fat in boys' diets were the higher values in all cases where data were given separately)

Figure 5.3 Proportions of food energy from fat

Comparison between a group of Asian infants and young children in Sheffield and a predominantly white population of the same age

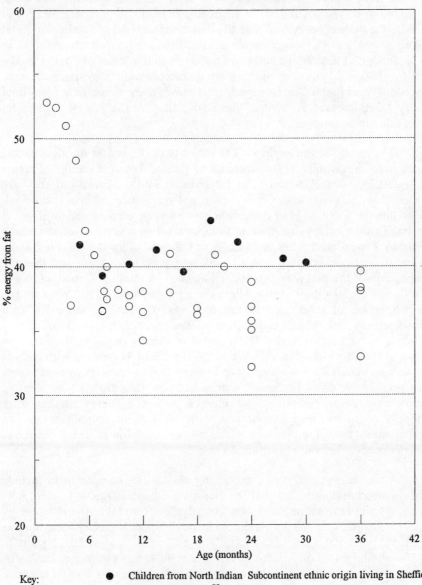

Key:

● Children from North Indian Subcontinent ethnic origin living in Sheffield
Fieldwork: 1989-90 [50]

○ data from 6 studies of British children who were predominantly white
(same as figure 5.2)

5.3.4 *Dietary fat and cardiovascular disease*   The report from COMA on Nutritional Aspects of Cardiovascular Disease[4] recommends that the population aged 5 years and older should consume no more than about 35 per cent of calories from fat and about 10 per cent of calories from saturated fatty acids. Children under 5 years of age are not included in this recommendation. The evidence, discussed in the COMA report, which links dietary fat in early years to the risk of cardiovascular disease in adult life is incomplete[51,52,53,54]. Growth in infancy and young childhood must be safeguarded because it signifies nutritional adequacy and also because poor growth has been associated with increased risk of ill health in adult life[55] (para 12.3). Fat provides the major energy source in the diet of infants and any reduction in fat is likely to give a diet of lower energy density. Increased carbohydrate intake in the weaning diet appears to compensate for declining levels of energy intake from fat (Figure 5.1). Although there are no recommendations specific for the pre-school years in the COMA report[4], it is sensible when moulding pre-school dietary habits to take account of the advice that by the age of 5 years fat intakes should be moderated.

5.3.5 *Cow's milk for under-fives*   The majority of dietary fat during weaning comes from breast milk, infant formula or unmodified cow's milk[10]. Parents may question when they can offer fat reduced milks especially if they are consumed in the household. Cow's milk is not recommended as a main drink during infancy (para 9.4) but during the second year, used as a main drink, it can make an important contribution to the intakes of several nutrients as well as energy. Fat reduced milks are usually unsuitable before the child is 2 years old because of concern that energy intakes may be inadequate and that the composition of the diet may become unbalanced. A study of Canadian babies aged 0 to 18 months showed that where the milk was reduced to 2 per cent fat, the proportion of solid food in the diet was significantly increased with unsatisfactorily high protein and sodium intakes[56]. A very low intake of dietary fat may also be a factor in the development of chronic non-specific diarrhoea known as "toddler's diarrhoea"[57]. When the records of 44 children with chronic non-specific diarrhoea, for whom 24 to 72 hour dietary histories were available were reviewed[58], many of these children had low (less than 17 per cent of dietary energy) or "marginal" fat intakes, although energy intakes were generally adequate. Supplementation with fat rich in polyunsaturates to approximately twice the previous intake was successful in relieving diarrhoea in 82 per cent of the children within 2 weeks.

5.3.6   After the age of 2 years the young child's diet may begin to include semi-skimmed milk provided that the diet is varied and adequate to meet fully the energy and nutrient needs. As the contribution from fat to the total energy requirements reduces, the deficit should be made up with starchy foods such as bread, potatoes, pasta and rice. A study of 153 children aged 2 to 5 years in Edinburgh found that there were no significant differences in energy intakes or growth rates between groups of children of the same age who derived less than 30 per cent, or who derived more than 40 per cent of energy from fat[59] (Annex I). Energy intake deficits in the low fat intake group were made up by increased carbohydrate intakes. The maintenance of adequate energy intakes must be paramount in determining the composition of the diet at these ages.

Many children's dietary habits are capricious and where there are doubts about the adequacy of energy and nutrient intakes whole cow's milk should continue to be used until the child is more readily accepting a diverse diet. Skimmed milk is not recommended before the age of 5 years.

5.3.7 *Long chain polyunsaturated fatty acids* Brain growth is rapid during the third trimester of pregnancy and the first year after birth when it accounts for 10 per cent of total body weight and it utilises 60 per cent of total energy intake. Brain and other neural tissue, including the retina, are largely composed of phospholipids which are rich in long chain polyunsaturated fatty acids (LCPUFA) especially docosahexaenoic acid and also arachidonic acid. Adults can synthesise these LCPUFAs from the essential fatty acids linoleic acid and alpha-linolenic acid obtained from the diet. The fetus cannot synthesise LCPUFAs and relies on an efficient transfer from the mother across the placenta and, after birth, from breast milk[60].

5.3.8 The enzymes required to synthesise LCPUFAs are inactive during fetal life and the capacity to convert essential fatty acids to LCPUFAs matures during the first half of infancy. This mechanism is not always efficient and infants who are fed current infant formulae incorporate alternative LCPUFAs, particularly those derived from linoleic acid, and have reduced amounts of docasahexaenoic acid in the brain[61]. Synthesis of LCPUFAs requires adequate amounts of both essential fatty acids in appropriate relative concentrations to act as substrate. The European Commission has proposed amendments to the Directive on Infant Formulae and Follow-on Formulae to require the addition of linoleic acid and alpha linolenic acid within specified limits. These additions, while ensuring adequate amounts of substrate, do not overcome the limited capacity of the immature pre-term infant, and to some extent also the term infant, to synthesise LCPUFAs.

5.3.9 The extent to which term infants are unable to synthesis LCPUFAs is uncertain. Circumstantial evidence on phospholipid brain composition suggests that synthesis of docosahexaenoic acid only becomes fully efficient after the first 4 months of life[61]. Evidence is accumulating that LCPUFAs are important in neuro-developmental development and visual cortical function[62,63,64,65]. By the time of weaning, healthy infants are probably able to meet their needs for long chain polyunsaturated fatty acids provided there is adequate dietary supply of essential fatty acid precursors. The quantities and qualities of dietary fats required to ensure healthy growth and development of infant tissues and organs, especially the vascular and the central nervous system, are the subject of much current debate and research. The long term implications for health and development need urgent investigation.

5.4 Carbohydrates

The Working Group recommends that

- **for groups of children the average intake of non-milk extrinsic sugars should be limited to about ten per cent of total dietary energy intake (para 5.5.2);**

- **provided energy intake is adequate, the proportion of energy supplied as starch in the weaning diet should increase as the proportion derived from fat decreases (para 5.6);**

- **the effects on nutritional status of high intakes by young children of foods which are rich in non starch polysaccharide and also often contain high phytate levels, should be evaluated (para 5.7.2).**

5.4.1 Carbohydrates have a wide range of chemical and physical structures and properties. Sugars are soluble carbohydrates, principally monosaccharides such as glucose, fructose and galactose, or disaccharides such as sucrose, lactose and maltose. Starches are alpha-glucan polysaccharide chains with diverse physical states capable of modification by procedures such as cooking. Non-starch polysaccharides (NSP) form a complex group of polymers derived largely from plant cell walls and identified by a specific enzymatic chemical method[66] and are the main constituents of "dietary fibre". NSP should supplant the term "dietary fibre" because it is more precise.

5.5 Carbohydrates: Sugars

5.5.1 *Dietary sugars* The COMA Panel on Dietary Sugars and Human Disease[67] classified sugars in foods as either intrinsic or extrinsic. *Intrinsic sugars* are naturally integrated into the cellular structure of a food. The most important sources are whole fruits and vegetables containing mainly fructose, glucose and sucrose. *Extrinsic sugars* are not located within the cellular structure of a food, they are either free in food or added to it. They include added sugars (recipe and table sugars) and sugars in fruit juices and honey. Extrinsic sugars are further classified as:

- *milk sugars* (mainly lactose) naturally occurring in milk and milk products,

- *non-milk extrinsic sugars (NME)* exclude the sugars in milk but include all other extrinsic sugars.

5.5.2 The milk sugar lactose contributes about 37 per cent of the energy in breast milk. Most infant formulae contain lactose only, but other carbohydrates such as sucrose, maltose and maltodextrins are permitted[45]. Sugars at ages 15 to 24 months contributed 26 to 29 per cent of total dietary energy, of which NME sugars formed a little over half[67]. The MAFF study found that at age 6 to 9 months sugars contributed 33 per cent of energy (9 per cent of energy from NME sugars), and 29 per cent of energy at age 9 to 12 months (12 per cent from NME sugars)[10]. The current UK recommendation is that for groups of people the intake of non-milk extrinsic sugars should contribute no more than an average of about 10 per cent of total dietary energy. This level is intended for the general population and it is based on a goal of reduced dental caries[28]. The Working Group considers that this value is applicable to preschool children, who are a group at high risk of dental caries.

5.5.3 *Sugars in the weaning diet* Sugars provide energy but they make no other contribution to overall nutrient needs. They can increase the palatability of food but they should be used sparingly. Most infants enjoy the taste of sweet foods (para 3.4) and small amounts may be helpful to improve the acceptance of foods such as desserts or stewed fruits, or a smear of jam may be used if the infant is otherwise reluctant to eat bread. During weaning it is important that the diet should offer a variety of tastes and textures and infants should not come to expect that their food and drink will always be sweet. Unsweetened cereals and yoghurts should be encouraged in preference to those containing sugars. There is no advantage to dental health if sucrose is replaced by other sugars or fermentable carbohydrate sweeteners such as honey, fruit juices or fructose.

5.6 Carbohydrates: Starch

5.6.1 The COMA Panel on DRVs concluded that, for the population as a whole, about 37 per cent of dietary energy should come from starch but recognised that for children aged under 2 years this value might be inappropriate[28]. The weaning diet should, as a priority, ensure adequate energy, and this is not easily provided by a starch rich diet which tends to be bulky although starch itself is well tolerated and efficiently absorbed (para 3.2.5). Cooked cereal products and vegetables provide suitable sources of starch in the weanling's diet and rice starch is well absorbed[68] and is particularly suitable during early weaning because it is gluten-free. Data on starch intakes by infants and young children are scarce since the few dietary surveys in this age group have usually reported total carbohydrate consumption with no distinction between sugars and starches. Two recent dietary surveys of young children reported considerable variation between children in the amount of starch consumed. The average daily intake of starch rose from 18 per cent of total energy at 6 to 12 months[10] to 21 per cent (girls) and 23 per cent (boys) at 4 years[69]. This trend to increasing starch intakes with age should be encouraged provided total energy intakes remain adequate.

5.7 Carbohydrates: Non-Starch Polysaccharides (NSP) "Fibre"

5.7.1 The recommendations of the COMA Panel on DRVs concerning NSP were limited to adults because there were insufficient data on the physiological effects of NSP in children[28]. Foods which are rich in NSP are not unsuitable during weaning providing they do not displace the more energy rich foods which children under two years need for growth. Infants and young children who receive diets inappropriately rich in low energy density foods may not get an adequate energy intake[70,71] which can result in failure to thrive[72] (para 12.2). Furthermore, a diet with too much NSP rich food if given to infants can cause diarrhoea.

5.7.2 Older infants and young children enjoy fruit and vegetables especially as snacks, and foods that are rich in NSP are often good sources of micronutrients. However, many foods rich in NSP such as cereal products and legumes also contain high levels of phytates which impair the absorption from the diet of divalent cations including, iron and zinc (para 7.3, 8.7) as well as some vitamins, although the clinical relevance of this is unclear. These relationships should be investigated further. The Working Group endorsed the view of the COMA Panel on DRV that the diets of children under 2 years should not contain NSP rich foods (especially those with high phytate levels) to the extent that the energy content of the diet or the bioavailability of micronutrients are compromised.

6. Vitamins and the weaning diet

The Working Group recommends that

- adequate vitamin status should be encouraged for mother and baby through a varied diet and moderate exposure to summer sunlight;

- foods and drinks which provide good sources of vitamin C should be encouraged in the weaning diet (para 6.3.3);

- breastfed infants under six months do not need vitamin supplementation provided the mother had an adequate vitamin status during pregnancy. From age six months, infants receiving breast milk as their main drink should be given supplements of vitamins A and D (para 6.6.2);

- infants fed on manufactured milks do not need vitamin supplements provided their consumption of infant formula or follow on milk is more than 500 ml per day. If they are consuming infant formula or follow on milk in smaller amounts or they are being given cow's milk, vitamins A and D supplements should be given (para 6.6.2);

- between the ages of one to five years, vitamins A and D supplements should be given unless adequate vitamin status can be assured from a diverse diet containing vitamins A and D rich foods and from moderate exposure to sunlight (para 6.6.2);

- research should be encouraged on the biological functions of the antioxidant vitamins C and E and the carotenoids, their turnover, requirements in childhood and the possible benefits or detrimental effects of high intakes (paras 6.1.4, 6.3.2, 6.5.1).

6.1 Vitamin A

6.1.1 Vitamin A is required for growth and for the development and differentiation of tissues. It is obtained from animal products in the diet as preformed retinol, or is made from certain of the carotenoids, in particular beta-carotene, in plant foods. Vitamin A activity, whether as preformed retinol or from carotenes, is expressed in retinol equivalents whereby 6 µg of beta-carotene is conventionally accepted to be nutritionally equivalent to 1 µg retinol in the range of foodstuffs provided by a mixed diet.

6.1.2 During weaning the major source of vitamin A in the diet is milk or infant formula. The vitamin A content of human milk is influenced both by the maternal diet during lactation and by the size of the mother's stores of this vitamin[73]. Breastfed infants do not show signs of vitamin A deficiency, even at intakes as low as 100 µg/d[74], although these levels would probably not be enough to ensure that the infant maintains satisfactory reserves. The RNI of 350 µg retinol equivalents per day should meet the needs of all healthy infants[28], while allowing for building and maintenance of liver stores[75] (Table 6.1). Only a limited number of foods provide vitamin A and the distribution of intake levels in a population on a mixed diet is highly skewed[76]. Therefore, while the mean of intakes recorded in the MAFF study was about twice the RNI[10], a proportion of children may have had low intakes particularly if they were drinking only small amounts of milk or infant formula. For this reason vitamin supplements continue to be recommended to ensure that all infants and young children have an adequate intake (para 6.6). A daily dose of Department of Health Vitamin Drops provides 200 µg retinol equivalents (Annex V).

6.1.3 Infants and children are particularly sensitive to the adverse effects of either deficiency or excess of this vitamin. Xerophthalmia, the ocular manifestation of severe vitamin A deficiency, is a common cause of blindness amongst children in the Third World. Young child mortality is high in areas where clinical and subclinical vitamin A deficiency is common. Vitamin A supplementation of children in these areas has led to reduction in young child mortality from infectious disease[77]. Toxic effects with bone and liver damage may arise following single very large doses of retinol or from ingestion of excessive doses of supplements over a long period. The Working Group endorsed the DRV Panel's recommendation that daily intakes of retinol should not exceed 900 µg in infants and 1,800 µg in young children of one to three years of age[28].

6.1.4 *Carotenoids* Apart from their pro-vitamin A activity, carotenoids have other important biological effects which are not shared by vitamin A. Beta-carotene is involved in maintaining an effective immune response[78]. Several carotenoids including beta-carotene appear to act as important antioxidants in tissues, together with vitamin C (para 6.3), vitamin E (para 6.5) and selenium (para 8.9), by deactivating or scavenging free radicals and activated oxygen, and might therefore protect against cellular damage[79] although further research is needed. There is insufficient evidence to quantify optimal intakes of each carotenoid and no DRVs have been set for beta-carotene. Vegetables and fruit are rich sources of carotenoids, as well as several other nutrients. The consumption of these foods should be encouraged at all ages.

6.2 B vitamins

6.2.1 The COMA Panel on DRVs endorsed the compositional guidelines for infant formula from an earlier COMA expert Panel[36]. These provided a basis for setting DRVs for thiamin and vitamin B6 (Table 6.1) and a safe level of intake for pantothenic acid. The RNI for riboflavin was derived from the amount of riboflavin required to produce satisfactory biochemical status in previously riboflavin deficient, breastfed Gambian infants[80]. DRVs for folate were based on the amount needed by infant formula fed infants in order to achieve growth rates, weight gains and haemoglobin concentrations similar to breastfed infants. The LRNI for vitamin B12 was set at 0.1 µg/d since this represents the amount of vitamin B12 that cures megaloblastic anaemia when given to Indian infants receiving less than 60 ng/d from breast milk[81]. The RNI for vitamin B12 was, however, set at 0.3 µg/d representing the intake required to normalise methyl malonic acid excretion[82]. DRVs for niacin were set at the same level as for adults. The Panel did not set a DRV for biotin because evidence was limited, but agreed that intakes between 10 and 200 µg/d were both safe and adequate for all age groups.

6.2.2   The dietary intakes of B vitamins in the 1986 MAFF survey were all found to be adequate as judged against the DRVs[10]. An infant breastfed by a vegan mother receives low levels of vitamin B12 intake from the breast milk. Infants who are weaned on vegan diets are at risk of becoming deficient in vitamin B12 and riboflavin (para 11.2).

6.3   Vitamin C

6.3.1   Vitamin C is an anti-oxidant vitamin which is essential to prevent scurvy and to promote wound healing. It is particularly valuable in assisting the absorption of iron from vegetables and other non-haem sources. This is probably achieved by chelating with iron to form a soluble compound which readily releases iron to the intestinal mucosa.

6.3.2   The COMA Panel on DRVs adopted 25 mg vitamin C per day as the RNI for infants[28] (Table 6.1). They set RNIs for children by interpolating between this and the RNI of 40 mg calculated for adults. The Panel concluded that more research was needed to verify claims that intakes of vitamin C above those necessary to cure scurvy can protect against, or cure, various diseases, tissue damage or improve general health. The MAFF survey of 1986 found that average vitamin C intakes were generally above RNI levels and that the main contributory foods were fruit juice, commercial baby foods and infant formulae[10].

6.3.3   Vegetables and fruits are the best sources of vitamin C and parents should be educated about which foods contribute larger amounts. A diet with a diversity of plant foods both raw and cooked is recommended and this may include vitamin C fortified products such as instant mashed potato and vitamin C enriched fruit drinks. Vitamin C is highly labile, it is destroyed by several factors including light, heat and oxygen. To retain high vitamin C levels foods given as meals or snacks should be fresh and lightly cooked. If foods, such as stews and curries containing vegetables, have undergone prolonged cooking, the vitamin C concentration is reduced. Salads or fresh fruit, especially citrus, to accompany such dishes as particularly advised.

6.3.4   The enhancing effect of vitamin C on the absorption of iron, and probably also zinc, from a meal is dependent on the presence of adequate amounts of vitamin C[83]. This level of intake may not be easy to achieve for fussy eaters and vitamin C enriched fruit drinks may be useful to increase the content. To be effective the drink should be consumed with the meal.

6.4   Vitamin D

6.4.1   Vitamin D is naturally present in only few foods. It is also obtained through photosynthesis in the skin by the action of ultraviolet-B radiation from sunlight on 7-dehydrocholesterol. Vitamin D_3, thus formed, is converted in liver and kidney to the active metabolite 25-hydroxyvitamin D $(1,25(OH)_2D)$[76]. Vitamin D status of the newborn is largely determined by the vitamin D status of the mother with cord blood concentration about 80 per cent of the mother's plasma level[84]. If maternal vitamin D status is poor during pregnancy, the newborn also has low plasma concentration and low stores of 25-hydroxvitamin D. Supplementary vitamin D is advised during pregnancy to ensure that the mother supplies enough to her baby before birth (Annex V).

6.4.2   Children under 3 years are particularly vulnerable to poor vitamin D status because of demands resulting from the high rate at which calcium is being laid down in bone. Vitamin D RNI values from birth to age 2 years are given in Table 6.1. Breast milk contains little vitamin D and breastfed infants depend on their stores at birth and their exposure to sunlight to maintain satisfactory vitamin D status. Infant formulae are fortified with vitamin D and, provided adequate amounts are consumed, infants fed these products are unlikely to become depleted. During weaning the amounts of vitamin D in the diet are generally low[10]. Formulated manufactured baby milks and fortified commercial foods contribute to the intake of vitamin D as does fatty fish (sardines, herrings, tuna etc) if consumed. Eggs make a minor contribution. Recently there has been evidence that meat contains higher amounts of 25-hydroxyvitamin D than had previously been recognised (B Mawer personal communication). If confirmed, this will need to be taken into account when assessing how best to ensure good vitamin D status during weaning.

6.4.3   Vitamin D deficiency is a long standing risk in the UK. In infants it may be due to inadequate vitamin D status of the mother during pregnancy. After birth, the infant may receive a diet low in vitamin D. There may also be little opportunity for synthesis in the skin, either because it is winter time, or because the infant is kept indoors or, when outside, is covered thoroughly. A successful programme of prevention has included vitamin supplementation of the whole population of pregnant mothers and children under 5 years. Recommendations for supplementation with vitamins A and D are described in para 6.6. The supplement available under the Welfare Foods Scheme provides 7 µg/d[3] which is the RNI for children from age 7 months to 3 years.

6.4.4   Pregnant Asian mothers, especially those who eat no meat, whether living in the UK or in their country of origin, have a greater risk of vitamin D deficiency[85]. Asian infants and young children are also more at risk of vitamin D deficiency. Fifteen years ago plasma 25-hydroxyvitamin D concentrations of under 10 ng/ml were found in 40 per cent, and very low concentrations of under 5 ng/ml in 6 per cent of children aged 20 to 24 months from Asian families in Birmingham[86]. Preventive measures, such as vitamin supplements for pregnant women and children under 5 years, dietary education and advice about the benefits of moderate exposure to sunlight have since been effective in improving the vitamin status of Asian under-fives. Throughout the past decade the number of cases of clinical rickets in Asians in the UK has declined and, the incidence is now very low[87]. More recently, children fed strict vegan diets from Rastafarian families were also recognised as being at risk of rickets[88]. The combination of a restricted diet and pigmented skin, which may be less efficient at synthesising vitamin D, is associated with a higher risk of vitamin D deficiency (Para 11.2) and several ethnic minority groups may be at risk.

6.4.5   High intakes of vitamin D can be toxic at all ages, and infants are especially vulnerable[36]. The COMA Panel on DRVs noted reports of hypercalcaemia arising from vitamin D intakes of 50 µg/d and mild hypercalcaemia was found in infants receiving 15 mg vitamin D orally every 3 to 5 months[89].

6.4.6   Care is also needed to ensure that exposure of skin to summer sunlight does not lead to sunburning which has been linked to an increased risk of developing malignant melanoma 20 to 30 years later[90]. Infants and young children are particularly at risk as are people of all ages who have pale skins. Infants and young children should not be placed in direct sunlight, where they may be at risk of sunburn in as little as 15 minutes at midday in the summer. Exposure at lower sun intensity would be preferred and prams should be placed in shade. Synthesis of vitamin D in the skin is highly efficient and no more than moderate exposure of lower arms, legs and face for 30 minutes a day during the summer is probably sufficient at UK latitudes. Sunbathing is not required.

6.5   Vitamin E

6.5.1   Tocopherols prevent propagation of the oxidation of unsaturated fatty acids by trapping free radicals. The most active component of vitamin E is alpha-tocopherol. Vitamin E inhibits the oxidation of long chain polyunsaturated fatty acids in phospholipids and defends vascular endothelial, neuronal and other cell membranes against damage from free radicals. This protective system is supported by peroxidase enzymes such as glutathione peroxidase[91]. Other nutrients involved in this protective system are vitamins A and C. Alpha-tocopherol appears to act synergistically with beta-carotene (para 6.1), the former is more effective at high, whilst the latter is more effective at low partial pressures of oxygen in reducing lipid peroxidation[92]. The minerals selenium, copper, zinc, iron and manganese also affect the rates of oxidation of unsaturated fatty acids and the release of prostenoids. The biological contributions of these nutrients to preventing oxidative damage should be investigated further.

6.5.2   No RNI was set for vitamin E, instead the dietary requirements are expressed in relation to the dietary intake levels of polyunsaturated fatty acids[28]. There is no recognised clinical syndrome of vitamin E deficiency in normal children. Children with severe and chronic fat malabsorption, for instance those with cystic fibrosis, may develop severe neurological disorders which can be prevented by vitamin E[93]. Vitamin E is widely available from the diet including human milk and also infant formulae to which it is added during manufacture.

6.6 Supplements of vitamins A and D

6.6.1 Satisfactory vitamin status during pregnancy and lactation helps to ensure the mother remains in good health and that she provides vitamin stores for her baby. It has long been recommended that all pregnant and lactating women and children under 5 years take dietary supplements of vitamins A, D and C. This has been regarded as so important that appropriate vitamin preparations have been made available at very low cost to all, with arrangements for free supplies for those in financial hardship (Annex V).

6.6.2 The advice about which groups of infants and children should be given vitamin supplements takes account of several factors. All infants should receive vitamin supplements with the following exceptions. Babies being breastfed who are thought likely to have good vitamin stores because the mother was in good vitamin status during pregnancy, may delay starting supplementation until aged 6 months. Where there is any doubt about the mother's vitamin status, supplementation should begin at age 1 month. Bottle fed infants who are consuming 500 ml infant formula or follow-formula a day do not need vitamin supplementation because these manufactured products are fortified with vitamin D. From age 1 year all young children should be given supplements to provide a safeguard at a time when it is difficult to be certain that the diet provides a reliable source. Vitamin supplements should be continued to the age of 5 years unless the child's diet is diverse and plentiful.

6.6.3 Infants and children at high risk of vitamin deficiency should particularly be encouraged to take supplements throughout the first 5 years. At risk groups include children living in more northerly latitudes of the UK, children from traditional Asian or Islamic communities, children born with poor stores of vitamin D including preterm infants, and children who are poor eaters and who consume only a limited number of foods. Children on restricted diets of choice such as vegan or macrobiotic diets as well as diets which exclude food items for the management of allergy or other disorders should particularly be advised to continue vitamin drops to age 5 years.

Table 6.1 *Reference Nutrient Intakes for vitamins for children aged less than 3 years*[28]

Vitamin	Age Group				
	0-3 months	4-6 months	7-9 months	10-12 months	1-2 years
Vitamin A (retinol equivalent) µg/d	350	350	350	350	400
Thiamin per 1000 kcal/d	0.3	0.3	0.3	0.3	0.4mg
Riboflavin mg/d	0.4	0.4	0.4	0.4	0.6
Niacin mg/d (mg niacin equivalent per 1000 kcal)	6.6	6.6	6.6	6.6	6.6
Vitamin B6 µg per g protein/d	8	8	10	13	15
Vitamin B12 µg/d	0.3	0.3	0.4	0.4	0.5
Folate µg/d	50	50	50	50	70
Vitamin C mg/d	25	25	25	25	30
Vitamin D µg/d	8.5	8.5	7	7	7

7. Iron and the weaning diet

The Working Group recommends that

- dietary sources of minerals should be provided by offering a variety of foods. Vitamin C in adequate amounts should be ensured with meals to assist absorption and this is particularly important if the diet is meat free (para 6.3). Continued use of iron-enriched infant formula or a follow on milk as a main drink after the first year should be considered if there are concerns about the adequacy of iron in the diet (para 7.3.2);

- immediate and long-term effects of iron deficiency with and without anaemia during weaning on health and development should be defined more precisely (para 7.2.4);

- there should be further investigation of the relationship between iron status and the quality and quantity of dietary intakes of iron including the extent to which iron fortified milks and foods contribute absorbable iron (para 7.3);

- means of preventing iron deficiency through effective nutrition education should be investigated further (para 7.4.1);

- laboratory criteria for anaemia and for iron deficiency should be defined and used to determine the prevalence of anaemia and of iron deficiency in the general population of children under two years of age in the UK (para 7.1.2, para 7.5);

- there should be an assessment of the need for universal or population sub-group screening for iron deficiency anaemia in infants and young children and for the feasibility and acceptability of such a programme (para 7.5);

- the natural history of iron deficiency in infants and young children in this country should be determined (para 7.5.5);

- the best method of intervention and follow-up of populations of young children who have been screened for iron status should be determined (para 7.5.5).

7.1 Anaemia and iron deficiency during weaning

7.1.1 In the United Kingdom iron deficiency is the most commonly reported nutritional disorder during early childhood and similar problems have been reported from other countries[94]. The high prevalence of anaemia reported from studies of British toddlers[95,86,96,97,98,99,100,101,50,11] is shown in Table 7.1 (World Health Organisation definition of anaemia : haemoglobin < 110 g per l[103]). Low serum ferritin concentration (< 10 µg per l) was even more

37

common although this measure cannot be used alone to define iron deficiency because it is influenced by other factors such as inflammation (para 7.5.3).

7.1.2   Studies in this country have examined populations from inner city areas or from Asian communities thought to be at high risk. There are no data about the haemoglobin and iron status in the general population of children under 2 years. The National Diet and Nutrition Survey commissioned by the Departments of Health and the Ministry of Agriculture, Fisheries and Food, examined a sample of children aged 1½ to 4½ years in 1992/3 who had been selected to be nationally representative of the population of Britain (para 2.3). Preliminary results show that 12 per cent of children were anaemic in the group aged 1½ to 2½ year and 6 per cent in both the 2½ to 3½ year group and the 3½ to 4½ year group using the WHO classification[11]. The proportions of children in the same three age groups who had a serum ferritin below 10 µg/l were 28 per cent, 18 per cent and 15 per cent respectively (Table 7.1). These values show that anaemia and iron deficiency are common in 2 year olds in this country and these conditions become less common as the children get older. Similar information should be obtained from a nationally representative group of under 2 year olds in this country.

Table 7.1   *Prevalence of anaemia (haemoglobin < 110g/l) and iron deficiency (serum ferritin < 10 µg/l) in infants and young children in Britain (based on a table by Stevens[102])*

Year of survey fieldwork	Location of survey	No subjects	Age (months)	Ethnic group	Proportion anaemic (%)	Proportion low serum ferritin (%)
1983/4[95]	Bradford	598	6-48	European	12	28
				Asian	28	45
1983[86]	Birmingham	134	21-23	Asian	31	57*
1984/5[96]	Birmingham	470	17-19	European	18	47**
				Asian	27	
1985[97]	Nottingham	130	15-24	European	16	Not
				Asian	26	estimated
				Caribbean	20	
1987/8[98]	London	148	8-24	European	17	Not
				Asian	26	estimated
				Predominantly Caribbean	18	
1988[99]	Newcastle	71	9-15	'Affluent'	11	Not
		70		'Deprived'	16	estimated
1988/9[100,101]	Bristol	122	12-24	European	18	Not
				Caribbean	25	estimated
1989/90[50]	Sheffield	138	4-40	Asian	11	34
1992/3[11]	Britain	300	18-29	Nationally representative	12	28
	Britain	353	30-41	Nationally representative	6	18

*   Percentage of total group with serum ferritin concentration < 7 µg/l.
** Percentage of anaemic children with serum ferritin concentration < 7 µg/l.

7.2 Clinical effects of iron deficiency in the first two years of life

7.2.1 Iron is a component of haemoglobin, of myoglobin, and of several enzymes. Iron deficiency can cause apathy and reduced exercise capacity. Young children who are affected often have poor appetites and this compounds the difficulty of improving iron status by dietary means. Some infants and young children with iron deficiency anaemia may appear happy and healthy and it is likely that they will remain undiagnosed. Once iron status is improved, usually by oral iron supplements, low haemoglobin and other haematological abnormalities quickly return to normal and mood improves in those children who had been listless.

7.2.2 Iron deficiency anaemia in toddlers is also associated with psychomotor delay. It is not certain whether this adverse effect is fully reversible with iron treatment[104]. Young North American children with iron deficiency anaemia showed a good response to a few days treatment with intramuscular iron with a significant increase in mental development indices on the Bayley scales of infant development[105]. Iron therapy for 2 to 3 months has been shown to improve psychomotor development in anaemic toddlers in two double blind randomly allocated placebo controlled trials. In this country, oral iron with vitamin C, or vitamin C alone, were given for 2 months to children aged 18 months with iron deficiency anaemia. Compared to the control group, significantly more of the iron and vitamin C group achieved the expected rate of psychomotor development and their rate of weight gain was greater[96]. In Indonesia, the effect of iron supplementation for 3 months on the Bayley scores of psychomotor development in a group of iron deficient anaemic children and in a group of non anaemic iron deficient children aged 12 to 18 months was compared in a placebo controlled trial with a group of non iron deficient, non anaemic children. Pre-treatment there were no differences in the developmental scores between the iron deficient non anaemic and the non iron deficient non anaemic groups. There was a significant difference between the scores of these two groups and the mean psychomotor scores of a group of iron deficient anaemic children. Iron therapy restored psychomotor deficits in the iron deficient anaemic group and this was not seen in the placebo treated group[106]. A field study in Costa Rica showed that the psychomotor performance of anaemic children was below that of non anaemic ones but improved significantly in those whose anaemia was corrected during 3 months of iron treatment. However, this was not a rigorous controlled trial[107].

7.2.3 There is evidence that deficits in psychomotor development associated with iron deficiency anaemia may not be fully reversible in the longer term in spite of treatment. In Chile a longitudinal study of children tested and treated for iron deficiency at one year of age found that lower mental development scores persisted at the most recent testing at 5 years of age[108]. Likewise, Costa Rican children with iron deficiency anaemia in infancy had increased risk of developmental deficit at 5 years[109]. The risk of permanent developmental deficits may be related to the duration of iron deficiency anaemia or to the child's age at the time of the deficiency[110]. The degree of iron deficiency is also likely to determine whether there is risk of permanent adverse effect.

7.2.4 These studies confirm an adverse effect of iron deficiency anaemia on psychomotor development. Iron treatment reverses haematological abnormalities and has been shown to reverse developmental delays when measured up to 3 months after a course of iron supplementation. However there may be long term effects which may not be wholly reversible although studies so far have extended only to the early school years. The immediate and long-term effects of iron deficiency in infants and young children in this country on health and development should be investigated further.

7.3 The causes of iron deficiency in young children

7.3.1 Babies born at term have accumulated iron in the liver and reticulo-endothelial tissues. Babies born pre-term do not have these stores of iron and are particularly vulnerable to deficiency during the first year. In addition, as a normal physiological response to post-natal life, the high haemoglobin level of the newborn falls and the iron thus liberated provides a further store for later months. There is little increase in body iron during the first four months of life (about 250 mg total at birth and at 4 months) but thereafter the total body iron increases to about 420 mg at the age of one year[111]. Iron is needed to meet this increasing requirement as well as to replace normal daily losses.

7.3.2 *Diet and iron deficiency during weaning* The major cause of iron deficiency in this age group is dietary although there are other factors. The level of iron in human milk is low but since about 50 per cent or more is absorbed, which is a high rate of absorption for iron, this makes an important contribution for the breastfed infant during early weaning. Lactoferrin, which constitutes 10 to 20 per cent of human milk protein, binds with two molecules of ferric iron to facilitate absorption via specific intestinal receptors. Bovine lactoferrin is not effective in this way and the efficiency of absorption of iron from cow's milk or from infant formula is much lower than from breast milk[112]. After the age of 6 months, the amount of iron contributed from breast milk is insufficient to meet increasing needs, and adequate intakes of iron, as well as of zinc and copper, must be ensured from other dietary sources. The absorption of iron from breast milk is greater if breast feeds are given separate from solid food. Solids given close to a breast feed reduce the bioavailability of iron from the breast milk because inhibitors in the food bind the iron from breast milk in unabsorbable complexes[113].

7.3.3 The measured iron content of a food does not necessarily reflect the amount which is absorbed when the food is eaten. Bioavailability describes the proportion of the total iron in a food, meal or diet that is utilised for metabolism. Iron is most readily absorbed from foods rich in haem, particularly red meat but also other meats and meat products. Non-haem iron, present in plants, is less well absorbed. Phytic acid from cereals, legumes and other vegetables, tannin in tea and polyphenols in spinach, coffee and to some extent, cocoa and herbs, all bind to iron, and hinder iron absorption[114]. Phosphoproteins present in cow's milk and in egg yolk bind with iron which further accounts for the limited absorption of iron from cow's milk. A wide range of foods commonly used during weaning prove to be poor sources of available iron.

7.3.4   It is a matter of concern that diets commonly used during weaning may provide inadequate absorbable iron. Foods containing haem iron should be introduced by 6 to 8 months (para 10.1) unless the infant is being weaning on a meat free diet. The absorption of iron and other minerals, such as zinc and copper, is enhanced by the presence in a meal of adequate vitamin C (para 6.3). Lightly cooked or raw vegetables and fruits are generally valuable components in the weaning diet including their contribution to vitamin C intake which assists the absorption of iron[115]. The presence of protein also increases iron absorption[116], possibly because protein combines with phytic acid in the upper intestine thus reducing its inhibitory effect on iron absorption. Foods poor in iron, such as cow's milk, should not be consumed as main foods until the mixed diet is well established and likely to provide adequate bioavailable iron from other sources. Breast milk or fortified infant formula or follow-on milk are therefore recommended in preference to cow's milk as the main drink before age 12 months (para 9.4). Foods which are known to inhibit iron absorption should be limited in amount especially where they make no significant contribution to the nutrient intake, such as tea and coffee (para 9.8). Infants on vegetarian weaning diets usually consume higher levels of phytates and particular care to avoid iron deficiency may be needed (para 11.2).

7.3.5   *Fortification of foods for infants and young children*   Fortification provides a means to increasing iron intakes from the diet (para 9.2, 9.3, 10.3). It is acceptable because consuming iron fortified foods appears to present no risks to children who already have satisfactory iron status. Iron fortification of manufactured "milks" and commercial baby foods reduces the prevalence of iron deficiency in groups who have been given these foods during weaning[117,115,118] although the scientific evidence is incomplete. Foods can be fortified with several iron salts but there are differences between individual iron compounds in their efficacy in providing a source of absorbable iron and in their storage life[119].

7.3.6   *Dietary intakes of iron during weaning in this country*   The MAFF survey in 1986[10] recorded the intakes of iron of older infants. The group aged 6 to 9 months had significantly greater intakes than infants aged 10 to 12 months. For both males and females in the younger group the mean and median intakes were above the RNI (Table 7.2). They had high intakes of fortified infant formulae and commercial infant foods. The iron intakes of the group aged 10 to 12 months were about 70 per cent of those of the younger group with mean and median intakes of both males and females below the RNI. Of this older group, 21 per cent had daily intakes below the LRNI (4.2 mg (74 µmol)). A factor associated with higher iron intakes was a diet containing larger amounts of infant formulae and commercial baby foods. Infants who were given mainly cow's milk and family foods tended to have lower iron intakes. Other UK *ad-hoc* studies have shown mean daily iron intakes of 8.8 mg (154 µmol) at 8 months and 5.8 mg (102 µmol) at 20 months[46] and 6.2 mg (109 µmol) at 6 to 12 months and 5.6 mg (98 µmol) at 1 to 2 years[48].

41

7.3.7   These low values for dietary iron intake are of concern because they are likely to be associated with an increased risk of iron deficiency and anaemia. Dietary recordings alone do not provide adequate information to assess iron status which can only be determined by blood analysis. There were no measures using blood analysis of iron status of the children in these studies.

7.3.8   *Blood loss from the gastro-intestinal tract*   It has been known for thirty years that some infants lose small amounts of blood from the gastro-intestinal tract but it is not clear whether this is pathological in all cases[120,121]. A recent study suggested that significant blood loss, calculated as equivalent to about a quarter of the iron absorbed, occurred in about a third of infants who from the age of 6 months had changed to whole cow's milk. Blood loss was less frequent in those given an infant formula[122]. The validity of methods used to assess faecal blood loss has been questioned[123]. In a similar, but not identical study significant blood loss was not confirmed[124]. This second study randomly assigned infants to receive cow's milk and iron fortified cereal or iron fortified infant formula or follow-on formula. The mean ferritin and mean corpuscular volume were lower at 12 months of age in the group receiving whole cow's milk and the proportion of children with very low plasma ferritin (<12µg/l) was

Table 7.2   *Reference Nutrient Intake values for iron up to 2 years of age(R) with mean and median iron intake levels (mg(µmol)) recorded between 6 and 12 months of age and the mean daily contribution from the foods providing a major source of iron*[10] *(Annex I).*

			Age group			
		0-3 months	4-6 months	7-9 months	10-12 months	1-2 years
RNI mg (µmol)/day		1.7 (30)	4.3 (80)	7.8 (140)	7.8 (140)	6.9 (120)
Daily dietary intake levels of iron						
male	mean			9.6 (168)	7.2 (126)	
	median			9.2 (161)	6.0 (105)	
female	mean			9.0 (158)	6.4 (112)	
	median			8.2 (144)	5.7 (100)	
Daily mean intake of iron from specified foods* (% total intake)						
infant formulae				2.0 (22%)	0.7 (10%)	
manufactured dried foods				2.4 (26%)	0.8 (12%)	
manufactured foods in tins or jars				1.3 (14%)	0.8 (13%)	
infant rusks				1.7 (18%)	1.0 (15%)	
breakfast cereals				0.5 (5%)	0.9 (13%)	

*   The foods listed contributed 10% or more of the total iron intake in either age group.

much higher in the whole cow's milk group (28 per cent) than in those receiving an infant formula or follow-on milk (<1 per cent). This was ascribed to the low availability of iron in the diet as a whole which consisted mainly of cereals[125].

7.4 The prevention of iron deficiency

7.4.1   Iron status of infants and young children can be improved through dietary modification, by the fortification of foods and by giving supplementary iron. Parents and others responsible for feeding toddlers should be advised about the risk of iron deficiency and the importance of preventing it by dietary means. They should be educated about which diets provide the most bioavailable iron sources, which food combinations enhance, and which reduce, the absorption of iron from foods. Educators and advisors need to be trained about how to prevent iron deficiency and how to ensure that contacts with parents are culturally sensitive. Even then, the rates of success in encouraging dietary improvements may be disappointingly low. A recent large scale study in Birmingham looking at the effect of dietary health education delivered by health visitors to mothers in the first year of life on the incidence of iron deficiency anaemia failed to show a decrease in anaemia or an increase in the dietary intakes of iron in the study group. Overall incidence in both study and control groups remained at 30 per cent (A Aukett – personal communication). More work is needed to identify means of effective nutrition education that will lead to preventing iron deficiency by dietary modification.

7.4.2   Iron supplements are used to treat iron deficiency and they have also been used to prevent it. Long term prophylactic iron supplements for infants and young children have been recommended in this country only in special circumstances, for instance, where the infant was born prematurely with low iron stores. There have been concerns about overdose of iron, about gastrointestinal disturbances resulting from high dietary intakes of iron and about the danger of poisoning if large doses are consumed accidentally. There is extensive North American experience of low dose iron supplementation with drops for infants and young children although supplementation probably offers no advantage when the diet contains iron fortified infant formulae[126]. Furthermore, iron supplementation of young children aged 12 to 18 months who were not iron deficient was associated with slower growth rates when compared with a group of iron replete young children who had not been supplemented[127].

7.5 Should there be a screening programme for anaemia?

7.5.1   Anaemia due to iron deficiency only presents clinically in a proportion of cases and blood analysis is necessary to identify all those affected. In suggesting in 1989 that a screening programme for anaemia in pre-school children should be considered, three questions were posed:

1. whether routine blood sampling would be acceptable to parents (and the children),

2. whether the incidence of iron deficiency anaemia could be reduced by appropriate health education,

3. what measurable benefits might result from a more aggressive approach to the identification and treatment of iron deficiency anaemia?[128]

7.5.2　There is still inadequate information to answer these questions but some progress has been made and further questions have been raised. If a screening programme is feasible, should it include all the population in this age group or should it be limited to particular groups identified as at high risk, such as those from ethnic minorities? Another practical issue questions the best age at which to screen for anaemia. Screening at age 12 months would coincide with a time of rapid neurological development and it also has the possible advantage of combining this procedure with Measles Mumps Rubella immunisation. However, 12 months of age may be too early to identify the peak prevalence of anaemia which appears to be between 20 to 24 months of age. A local screening programme in Bristol found several children who were normal at 12 months but who subsequently developed iron deficiency anaemia[129]. The most appropriate laboratory tests for screening for iron deficiency anaemia also need to be determined; finger prick sampling for haemoglobin and another criterion, such as ferritin, may be suitable. The feasibility of using absorbent paper to collect and transport a spot of blood for laboratory analysis is being assessed. If early tests are successful this should be evaluated in field studies. At the same time reference levels used to assess haemoglobin and iron status should be examined. Although values quoted earlier have been adopted widely (para 7.1), they are generally values extrapolated from adult standards and may not be the most appropriate cut-off levels to define anaemia and iron deficiency in infants and young children.

7.5.3　*The laboratory diagnosis of anaemia and iron deficiency*　Children who test positive in a screening programme for iron deficiency anaemia need further detailed evaluation to confirm the diagnosis. Iron status, is best determined from a combination of tests although which grouping gives the most accurate diagnosis in this age group remains uncertain and should be investigated. Haemoglobin concentration and blood film examination provide indirect evidence of iron status. Deficiency causes anaemia with hypochromia, microcytosis and anisocytosis but there are also other causes for these changes. Serum ferritin concentrations fall as iron stores become depleted. Levels of erythrocyte protoporphyrin indicate failure of incorporation of iron into haem. Determination of the iron binding capacity of the blood reflects the saturation of the iron-carrying protein molecules with iron; high levels imply poor iron status. These measurements are affected by factors apart from iron status, such as inflammation, hypoprotein aemia or haemoglobinopathies all of which cause difficulties in interpretation. There is also a degree of interference between different minerals such as zinc, iron and lead that bind the same proteins. A transferrin receptor assay has recently been developed and this needs to be evaluated. When iron balance is negative the serum iron falls and serum transferrin rises so that the transferrin saturation is considerably reduced. Techniques for blood analyses should be subject to adequate standards of quality control.

7.5.4   A strategy for managing children who have been screened should be developed. Those identified as iron deficient may need iron supplements or iron injections and there should be expert advice and support to achieve modification of the child's diet. Because of lack of information on the natural history of iron deficiency anaemia at this age, it is uncertain whether a single test is all that is needed. Should all of the group, or the iron deficiency group only, or none of the group be re-screened, and after what period? Further studies of the natural history of iron deficiency should be given priority.

8. Minerals (excluding iron) and the weaning diet

The Working Group recommends that

- there should be adequate dietary intake of calcium. For young infants the dietary calcium to phosphorus ratio should be between 1.2 and 2.0 by weight (0.9:1 to 1.6:1 (molar)) (para 8.1, 8.2);

- research should be encouraged on calcium, phosphorus and magnesium metabolism in children. The interactions of these nutrients together with factors which modulate them, including diet and the mechanisms for adapting to diets poor in these nutrients should be clarified (para 8.1.1, 8.2, 8.3);

- investigations should be encouraged to determine the optimal balance of iron, zinc and copper in the weaning diet (para 8.7.2, 8.8.2);

- research should be encouraged on the inter-relationship of vitamins C and E and the carotenoids with fatty acids, selenium, iron, zinc, copper and manganese on the levels of antioxidant activity in developing infant tissues (para 6.5.1, 8.8.1, 8.9).

8.1 Calcium

8.1.1 The vast majority of calcium in the body is found in the skeleton although this ion is also needed for the normal function of all cells. Its level is closely regulated by a variety of hormonal systems. The COMA Panel on DRVs assumed an absorption efficiency of calcium from breast milk of about 66 per cent, and from infant formula of about 40 per cent[28]. For children over the age of one year on a mixed weaning diet an absorption of 35 per cent has been assumed, although this value is largely based on data from adults. The EARs for calcium probably describe the apparent calcium requirements which have been derived by a number of techniques, such as retention or balance studies of healthy people in the UK consuming diets usual for this country, rather than a true basal dietary requirement (Table 8.1). The RNIs and LRNIs are based on the EARs by adding or subtracting 30 per cent, being 2 notional standard deviations. The RNIs for infants may be higher than that available from some formulae. The apparent requirements for calcium may be influenced by prevailing dietary habits. It is thought that there are mechanisms for adapting to diets low in calcium but they are, as yet, poorly understood. Positive calcium balances have been maintained in children on relatively low calcium diets although rickets and osteomalacia may result when intakes are very low[130]. More information is needed on calcium bioavailability and mechanisms to adapt to varying levels of calcium in the diet.

8.1.2   Milk and milk products provide the richest and most easily absorbed dietary sources of calcium, and products made from white flour which is fortified currently also make an important contribution. The consumption of milk by the nation as a whole has been declining steadily and this decline probably also affects young children (Table 8.2). In the MAFF survey, cow's milk and milk products, infant formula and breast milk together contributed about 65 per cent of calcium in diets which on average provided daily intakes of 783 mg, which is substantially above the RNI[10].

8.2   Phosphorus

8.2.1   Most phosphorus in the body is linked to calcium in the bones and teeth. Phosphorus has an essential role in energy release and other metabolic processes. It is present in phospholipids which are incorporated in neural tissue in early life and in all membranes (para 5.3). The RNIs for calcium and phosphorus have been set as equimolar (Table 8.1) which reflects their relative presence by weight in the body. There is risk of neonatal tetany related to hypocalcaemia and hyperphosphataemia[36] and therefore, for young infants, the ratio of dietary calcium to phosphorus should between 1.2 and 2.0 by weight (0.9:1 and 1.6:1 (molar)). The MAFF study showed that between 6 to 12 months of age 50 per cent of dietary phosphorus came from milk and that mean intake was 742 mg (24.3 mmol)/day[10].

8.3   Magnesium

8.3.1   Magnesium and calcium are mutually involved in several metabolic processes. Most magnesium in the body is in the skeleton and, next to potassium, it is the dominant intracellular cation. The interactions between calcium, phosphorus and magnesium are complex and not fully understood[36,130]. The RNI (Table 8.1) was exceeded in the diets of the infants in the MAFF study with a mean intake of 124 mg (5.1 mmol)/day at 6 to 12 months (R MAFF)[10].

8.4   Sodium

8.4.1   The COMA Panel on DRVs addressed sodium intake in terms of physiological requirements, but data for children during weaning are scarce. The LRNI for infants up to six months (140 mg (6 mmol)/day) approximates to intake values calculated for breastfed infants (850 ml milk per day, containing 165 mg (7 mmol)/l) (Table 8.1). The LRNI for children over 1 year has been estimated by calculating the daily increment (mainly in extracellular fluid) for growth, and allows for dermal, faecal and urinary losses[28].

8.4.2   Infants, as adults, are efficient at conserving sodium by reducing losses in the urine. They are less efficient than adults in excreting an excess and, for this reason, the sodium intakes of infants should be moderated (para 3.2). The sodium content of infant formulae is regulated to give levels of around 25-30 mg (1.1-1.3 mmol)/100 kcal. By the age of 4 months healthy infants increase their ability to excrete a sodium load. However, throughout weaning it is prudent to moderate dietary salt levels. This can be achieved by not adding salt to foods.

8.4.3   There is evidence that habitual sodium intakes in adult populations are a determinant of prevailing levels of blood pressure[131]. There is some evidence that levels of blood pressure in childhood "track" from the age of 2 years or more through to adulthood[3]. The nature of any relationship between sodium intake in the first few years of life and lifelong blood pressure levels is far from clear, but populations with low sodium intakes experience a lower rise in blood pressure with age[132]. Parents can help pre-school children towards a lifetime of healthy eating habits by reducing salty foods in their children's diets.

8.5   Potassium

8.5.1   Potassium is the major intracellular cation where it is maintained at a concentration of 5.7 g (145 mmol) per litre. An appreciable fraction of the energy required in the basal metabolic state is used for the exchange of sodium and potassium by active transport mechanism across cell membranes. This ensures that sodium is kept predominantly in the extracellular, and potassium in the intracellular compartments, thus regulating the extracellular fluid volume, the plasma and intracellular osmolarity, the acid base balance and the membrane potential of cells. The intracellular potassium concentration is more than thirty times the concentration found in plasma and interstitial fluid. The small percentage of extracellular potassium is of major importance in the transmission of neuronal messages, muscular contractility and the maintenance of normal blood pressures. Adequate potassium intakes are essential to maintain these processes. During infancy approximately 2.7 g (70 mmol) of potassium are required for each kilogram of weight gained. In addition to calculations based on increases in lean body mass there is obligatory urinary, cutaneous and faecal loss to take into account. An intake of 78 mg (2 mmol) per 100 kcal would maintain potassium balance in normal children.

8.5.2   Human milk contains about 600 mg (15 mmol) potassium per litre and levels in infant formulae are regulated to be similar, while cow's milk contains larger amounts, usually about 1,400 mg (35 mmol) per litre. The richest dietary sources are unprocessed foods, especially fruits, many vegetables and fresh meats. The MAFF survey showed that the mean dietary intakes of potassium in infants aged 6 to 12 months were well in excess of the RNI[10] (Annex I) (Table 8.1).

8.6   Chloride

8.6.1   Chloride is the principal inorganic ion in extracellular fluid and is essential for maintaining fluid and electrolyte balance and transmembrane potentials. It is also necessary for the production of hydrochloric acid in gastric juice and is therefore essential in food digestion. Its intracellular concentration is low and plasma and extracellular concentrations range from 3.4 to 3.8 g (96-106 mmol) per litre.

8.6.2   Dietary chloride is predominantly in the form of sodium chloride. The intake of chloride from food and losses from the body in urine, sweat and faeces are linked to that of sodium, therefore the requirements are similar to those of sodium. During the first year of life, however, as the relative demand for potassium is so great and potassium chloride is a dietary constituent, the chloride requirement is greater than during the rest of life. Human milk contains 450 mg (12.7 mmol) chloride per litre and a similar value is present in most infant formulae. This ensures a ratio of sodium plus potassium to chloride of 1.5 - 2.0 to maintain the requirements of acid base regulation[133]. The chloride intakes in children aged 6 to 12 months in the MAFF survey were fully adequate[10] (Table 8.1).

8.7   Zinc

8.7.1   A wide range of metabolic processes require zinc including nucleic acid synthesis and cell division. The clinical features of zinc deficiency are diverse and non-specific unless the deficiency is very severe as in acrodermatitis enteropathica. Zinc deficiency may limit growth velocity. Trials of zinc supplementation in infancy found that zinc supplemented groups gained weight and length more rapidly than control groups who were not supplemented although in both studies the infants were of poor socio-economic circumstances in the USA[134] and in France[135]. The dietary patterns of these infants are likely to differ substantially from diets in this country and these findings might not be repeated in children from more affluent homes.

8.7.2   The bioavailability of zinc is influenced by other dietary components. Inorganic iron may reduce the absorption of inorganic zinc especially when there is proportionately excess iron over zinc[136]. It is important that the iron content of infant formulae should not be increased unless it can be ensured that zinc availability remains adequate. Phytates form insoluble complexes with zinc and this is more pronounced if there is excess calcium in the diet. This raises the possibility that, as with iron, the introduction of weaning foods can reduce the efficiency of absorption of zinc.

8.7.3   For the purposes of defining RNIs, average zinc absorption from infant formulae and from mixed diets is assumed to be 30 per cent. Because zinc absorption increases at lower levels of zinc status, the COMA Panel on DRVs set the LRNIs based on a 50 per cent absorption efficiency in infants. Daily zinc requirements were then calculated factorially for infants. For children over the age of 1 year, RNIs were based on interpolated basal adult losses and calculated increments for growth, although these figures may be rather generous[28] (Table 8.1).

8.7.4   The 1986 MAFF survey found that the average daily zinc intake of infants aged 6 to 8 months was 4.3 mg (64.5 mmol) which was also the median value, and for infants aged 9 to 12 months the average intake was 4.8 mg (72 mmol) per day (median 4.6 mg (69 mmol))[10]. The RNI for this age group is 5 mg (75 mmol) per day. Six per cent of infants had daily zinc intakes below the LRNI (3 mg (45 mmol)/ day). The contribution to total zinc intakes from breast milk, infant formula and cow's milk was significant because, although zinc concentrations in these foods are low, they were major dietary components. Meat and meat products are the richest dietary sources of zinc, but these foods contributed only 10 per cent of the dietary zinc intake. Although nearly 70 per cent of infants in this study were eating meat, the quantities were small. In 1990, the infant feeding survey recorded that 94 per cent of infants ate meat at least once a week by the age of 9 months, and 40 per cent ate meat every day[9]. In spite of this frequent consumption of meat the level of zinc intake was scarcely adequate in the MAFF study and parents may need to be encouraged to give their infants larger servings of meat.

8.8 Copper

8.8.1   Copper is involved in cell and tissue growth, is a co-factor with a number of metalloproteins including cytochrome oxidase and superoxide dismutase which are essential for oxidative metabolism, and is involved in nerve myelination and in the metabolism of several steroid hormones[28]. The effects of copper deficiency may include loss of muscle strength, bone defects, disorders of the central nervous system, hypopigmentation, impaired growth and anaemia.

8.8.2   Clinical copper deficiency during infancy in babies who were born pre-term is a recognised hazard[137]. Infants born at term have a liver store of about 8 mg (130 µmol) copper and this protects them from any apparent growth or health differences even where dietary copper intakes are low[138]. Human milk is a good source of copper although the concentration declines from about 4 months. It has been questioned whether the availability of copper from infant formula is reduced when iron or zinc concentrations are relatively increased. No deficiency of copper absorption was shown when infants were fed with infant formulae with high levels of iron fortification[139]. In spite of this reassurance, further information is needed on the immediate and longer term effects of the relative concentration of iron, zinc and copper in infant formulae. Once the infant is on a mixed diet, adequate intakes of copper from non-milk sources including green vegetables, cereals and meat are readily obtained.

8.8.3   There were insufficient data for the COMA Panel on DRVs to derive EARs or LRNIs for copper at any age. For infants, the requirements were calculated factorially and were interpolated for children from data available for specific ages[28].

8.9 Selenium

8.9.1   Selenium in human milk is present in the enzyme glutathione peroxidase which protects fat from peroxidation. The level of selenium in cow's milk is about one half of that in human milk and in spite of supplementing infant formulae based on cow's milk with selenium the absorption is less efficient than from human milk[140]. No adverse effects of lower levels of selenium intake from infant formulae have been observed in this country. However, in principle, any reduction in capacity to cope with oxidative stress at a time when the infant is consuming a high fat, high iron diet, may be undesirable.

8.10 Iodine

8.10.1 The MAFF survey of older infants found that iodine intakes substantially exceeded the RNI (60 µg (0.5 µmol)/d)[10] (Table 8.1). The mean daily intake in the group aged 6 to 8 months was 176 µg (1.5 µmol) and in the older group aged 9 to 12 months it was 235 µg (2 µmol). "Milks" contributed 70 per cent of iodine intake. The iodine content of cow's milk is higher than in human milk or infant formulae (Table 9.1). There is seasonal variation in iodine content in cow's milk which is ascribed mainly to differences in the iodine content of the cows' feed with iodine rich concentrates dominating the winter diet[141]. The MAFF study carried out during November used a value of 37 µg (0.3 µmol)/100 ml which is an average concentration for iodine in cow's milk in winter (level in summer milk is 7 µg (0.6 µmol)/100 l). However, using the lower summer value for milk, intakes would still exceed the RNI for this age group. There are no concerns about iodine deficiency during weaning.

Table 8.1   *Reference Nutrient Intakes for calcium, phosphorus, magnesium, sodium, potassium, chloride, zinc, copper, selenium, iodine for children less than 3 years*[28]

Nutrient	Age group				
	0-3 months	4-6 months	7-9 months	10-12 months	1-2 years
Calcium mg(mmol)/d	525 (13.1)	525 (13.1)	525 (13.1)	525 (13.1)	350 (8.8)
Phosphorus mg(mmol)/d	400 (13.1)	400 (13.1)	400 (13.1)	400 (13.1)	350 (8.8)
Magnesium mg(mmol)/d	55 (2.2)	60 (2.5)	75 (3.2)	80 (3.3)	85 (3.5)
Sodium mg(mmol)/d	210 (9)	280 (12)	320 (14)	350 (15)	500 (22)
Potassium mg(mmol)/d	800 (20)	850 (22)	700 (18)	700 (18)	800 (20)
Chloride mg(mmol)/d	320 (9)	400 (12)	500 (14)	500 (15)	800 (22)
Zinc mg(µmol)/d	4.0 (60)	4.0 (60)	5.0 (75)	5.0 (75)	5.0 (75)
Copper mg(µmol)/d	0.3 (5)	0.3(5)	0.3 (5)	0.3 (5)	0.4 (6)
Selenium µg(µmol)/d	10 (0.1)	13 (0.2)	10 (0.1)	10 (0.1)	15 (0.2)
Iodine µg(µmol)/d	50 (0.4)	60 (0.5)	60 (0.5)	60 (0.5)	70 (0.6)

Table 8.2   *Consumption of milk 1952-1993* (per person/week)*

Year	Liquid whole milk (pints)	Reduced fat milks (pints)	Total milk and cream† (pints)
1952	4.82	—	5.09
1962	4.95	—	5.26
1972	4.62	0.01	5.05
1977	4.54	0.02	4.90
1982	3.95	0.08	4.40
1987	2.88	0.78	4.07
1992	1.74	1.70	3.90
1993	1.58	1.81	3.83

* Source MAFF National Food Survey - Great Britain (provided per person for the total population; no separate data for infants and children).

† This group, as well as liquid cow's milk, includes also condensed milk, infant formula and instant milks.

9. Milk and other drinks

The Working Group recommends that

● breast milk provides the best source of nourishment for the early months of life. Mothers should be encouraged and supported in breastfeeding for at least four months and may choose to continue to breastfeed as the weaning diet becomes increasingly varied (para 9.1);

● an infant who is not breastfed should receive infant formula or follow-on milk. Follow-on milk is not recommended as replacement for breast milk or infant formula before six months (para 9.2, 9.3);

● pasteurised whole cow's milk should only be used as a main milk drink after the age of one year. Intakes of iron and zinc and vitamins A and D should be ensured from other dietary sources or from supplements. Semi-skimmed cow's milk is not suitable as a drink before the age of two years but thereafter it may be introduced gradually if the child's energy and nutrient intake is otherwise adequate and if growth remains satisfactory. Fully skimmed cow's milk should not usually be introduced before the age of five years (para 9.4);

● goat's and sheep's milks should not be given to infants, and if used after this age the milk must be pasteurised or boiled (para 9.5);

● milk (also including breast milk, infant formula, follow on formula) or water should constitute the majority of the total drinks given. Other drinks should usually be confined to meal times and because of the risk to dental health, they should not be given in a feeding bottle or at bedtime (para 9.2, 9.8).

9.1 Human milk

9.1.1 The nutrient composition of human milk was determined in a study of pooled milk samples which had been taken singly from 96 breastfeeding women in the UK at about 5 to 6 weeks post delivery[43]. The energy and nutrient levels of human milk from this study are listed in Table 9.1 as are the levels in cow's milk, and the levels in infant formula and follow-on formula in the European Directive[45] which governs the composition of these manufactured products. In assessing the energy and nutrient composition of human milk it is important to be aware that several factors cause variations. For instance, the fat concentration in the milk increases as the breast is emptied. The range and concentrations of fatty acids in milk are influenced by the mother's dietary intake which probably accounts for worldwide differences in the quality and quantity of fat in human milk[143] and the same is true for iodine and other micronutrients. Breast milk composition is also influenced by the stage of lactation.

9.1.2   The energy value for human milk of 70 kcal/100 ml reported from the study above is usually quoted as the standard but it may be too high, and more recent studies which take account of data from energy expenditure studies have suggested that the mean value lies between 60 and 70 kcal/100 ml[144,145]. The energy value of milk is mainly determined by its fat content which contributes about 50 per cent to the total energy of milk of women in the UK. The fat in human milk is well absorbed when compared with fats of non-human origin and this has been ascribed to its stereoisomeric structure[146]. Twenty to 25 per cent of human milk fat is palmitic acid and it is in the middle (sn-2) position of the triglyceride molecule which is associated with high rates of absorption. In non-human milk fats palmitic acid is more evenly distributed between the three positions on the triglyceride, a configuration which leads to less ready absorption by human infants. Efficient fat absorption is beneficial to ensure adequate energy from the diet. It also means that there are lower levels of free fatty acids in the gut to bind with dietary calcium as unabsorbable soaps. The loss of bioavailable calcium is particularly undesirable for preterm infants who commonly suffer metabolic bone disorders (para 11.3). Breast milk also provides balanced and adequate amounts of the essential fatty acids linoleic acid and alpha linolenic acid (para 5.3) as well as long chain polyunsaturated fatty acids for incorporation into brain and retina.

9.1.3   Human milk has less protein than other milks with a very low casein content. A high proportion of the whey fraction consists of immunologically active proteins such as alpha lactalbumin and lactoferrin which, as well as enabling the absorption of iron (para 7.3), also inhibits the growth of micro organisms. Passive transfer of immunoglobulin G and M from mother to infant in the milk is much less than in ruminants but breast milk cells contribute to defences against pathogenic organisms through the production of immunoglobulin A.

9.1.4   Lactose contributes about 37 per cent of the energy in human milk and levels are higher than in cow's milk (Table 9.1). Many micronutrients are more readily absorbed from breast milk than from the milk of other species or from manufactured formulae (para 7.3), so that even small quantities of breast milk can be a useful addition to the weaning diet. However, from six months of age, breast milk cannot supply the requirements for several micronutrients, particularly iron, copper and zinc, and alternative dietary sources should be ensured.

9.1.5   Breastfeeding offers the newborn the best nutrition. Apart from providing the most appropriate balance and concentration of nutrients, it offers them in a digestible form and there are also enzymes to assist with digestion. Milk has evolved to provide nourishment and protection during a vulnerable period of life. In Dundee, Scotland, babies who had received breast milk up to the age of 13 weeks had reduced risk of gastrointestinal and respiratory infections when compared with infants who had been given infant formulae, and this benefit persisted throughout the first year of life even after breastfeeding had ceased[147]. Breastfeeding is recommended for infants who have a family history of allergy (para 11.1) although the extent of protection provided by breastfeeding and the mechanisms involved remain unclear. One possible explanation is that babies being exclusively breastfed are prevented from contact with allergens in cow's milk[148]. Ideally the mother should also avoid likely allergens in her diet since many, including intact cow's milk protein, are secreted into the milk. There may also be benefits from reduced risk of gastro-intestinal disorders in later life such as Crohn's disease and coeliac disease although results from studies differ (para 12.3.5). It is advised that breastfeeding should continue for 4 months at least, and ideally, throughout the first year. Lactation may be tapered during the period of mixed feeding by giving other fluids.

Table 9.1   *Composition of human milk and cow's milk: compositional guidelines for infant formula and follow on formula (per 100ml)*

		Mean values for mature human milk[43]	Mean values for whole cow's milk[+]	Infant formula*	Follow on formula*
Energy	kJ	293	284	250-315	250-335
	kcal	70	68	60-75	60-80
Protein	g	1.3**	3.3	1.2-1.95	1.5-2.9
Carbohydrate	g	7	4.9	4.6-9.1	4.6-9.1
Fat	g	4.2	4.0	2.1-4.2	2.1-4.2
Vitamins					
A	μg(RE)	60	57	39-117	39-117
D	μg	0.01	0.03	0.65-1.63	0.65-1.95
E	mg(&TE)	0.35	0.09	≥0.33	≥0.3
K	μg	0.21	0.6	2.6	ns
Thiamin	μg	16	31	265	ns
Riboflavin	μg	30	175	39	ns
Niacin	μg	620	802	163	ns
equivalent***	μg	620	802	163	ns
B6	μg	6	62	22.8	ns
B12	μg	0.01	0.4	0.07	ns
Total folate	μg	5.0	6	2.6	ns
Panthothenic acid	μg	260	361	195	ns
Biotin	μg	0.8	2.0	1.0	ns
C	mg	3.8	1.0	5.2	5.2
Minerals					
Sodium	mg	15	57	13-39	ns
Potassium	mg	60	144	39-94	ns
Chloride	mg	43	103	32.5-81	ns
Calcium	mg	35	119	19.5	ns
Phosphorus	mg	15	95	16.3-58.5	ns
Magnesium	mg	3	11	3.3-9.8	ns
Iron	μg	76	62	325-975	650-1300
Copper	μg	39	tr	13-52	ns
Zinc	μg	295	412	325-975	325
Iodine	μg	7	15	3.3	3.3

+   data on nutrition levels in cow's milk provided by MAFF.

*   EC Directive The acceptable range (one value only indicates minimum permissable values) (see para 9.2)[45]. Calculated from EC Directive for a product containing 65 kcal/100ml.

**   True protein = 0.85 g per 100 ml (excludes non-protein nitrogen) although a proportion of the non-protein nitrogen is used for the maintenance and growth of infants[142].

***   Of this, 720 mg/100 ml is derived from tryptophan.

ns =   not specified.

tr =   trace.

9.2 Infant formula

9.2.1   Infant formulae are manufactured to provide a sole source of nourishment for young infants. Traditionally sold as dry powder to be reconstituted with water, ready to feed bottles and cartons of infant formula are now also available. Compositional guidelines for infant formula (whether based on cow's milk protein or on soya protein isolate) and for follow on formula have been agreed in 1991 in a European Commission Directive[45] (Annex II) and UK regulations to implement this Directive will come into force during 1994. The compositional requirements in the European Directive are defined on an energy basis. For the purpose of comparison with human and cow's milk compositions these values have been used to calculate the compositions of infant formula and follow on formula on a weight per 100 ml basis using products with 65 kcal/100 ml as typical (Table 9.1). It should be recognised that this introduces some distortion in that the ranges of protein, carbohydrate and fat are not as large as they appear from Table 9.1 when the product is considered as a whole.

9.2.2   In the manufacture of infant formulae the total protein concentration in cow's milk is reduced and, in some products, the overall proportion of casein is lowered. Casein dominant milks are based on whole cow milk protein and have a casein : whey ratio of approximately 80 : 20. Whey dominant milks are modified so that the cow's milk protein has a casein : whey ratio of approximately 40 : 60 which is similar to that of human milk. The carbohydrate most commonly used is lactose, also allowed are maltodextrin and glucose syrups which are partial hydrolysates of starch containing oligosaccharides, disaccharides and monosaccharides, such as glucose, in varying proportions. Constraints are defined in the European Directive on the fats in infant formulae and follow on formulae. A few fats and oils are prohibited, there are upper limits to the concentrations of lauric, myristic and erucic acids and the essential fatty acid linoleic acid is required within a permitted range[45]. The importance of alpha linolenic acid has long been acknowledged[36,142] and this essential fatty acid is now included in the formulae available in the UK. The question of whether infant formulae should also include long chain polyunsaturated fatty acids has recently been considered[149] (para 5.6.3).

9.2.3   The micronutrient composition of infant formula is designed to reflect mean values of human milk but there are important exceptions. The absorption of some micronutrients, particularly minerals, from infant formulae is generally less efficient than is their absorption from human milk (para 7.3). To overcome poor bioavailability, manufacturers increase the levels of specified minerals when compared with levels in human milk in the expectation that more may be absorbed if there are higher levels in the food. It is uncertain that "high iron" infant formulae are needed in the first 3 to 4 months of life[150] given the high levels of iron stores available at this time (para 7.3). The European Directive permits "low iron" infant formulae although in the United Kingdom all products currently retailed are fortified. Zinc levels are also raised above those in human milk although not as much as iron levels. Vitamin D levels in infant formulae are much higher than those in human or cow's milk to help to ensure that infants obtaining little from synthesis in the skin have an adequate supply from the diet, and supplementary vitamin drops provide a similar reassurance (para 6.6).

9.2.4 For infants who are not being breastfed, infant formula offers a satisfactory sole source of nutrition to age 4 to 6 months, and in the early stages of a mixed diet they continue to provide the majority of energy and nutrients. Breast milk and/or infant formula are advised as main drinks in the diet throughout the first year of life and may be continued for longer. Infant formulae offer good supplies of vitamin D and most are rich in iron.

9.3 Follow on formula

9.3.1 Follow on formulae are based on cow's milk, they are intended to provide a nutritious drink component in the diet but not to be used as a sole source of nutrition. The European Directive specifies fewer compositional criteria[45] (Table 9.1; Annex II). The levels of vitamin D and iron are higher than those in human or cow's milk with a minimum level of iron twice the specified minimum for infant formula, and most brands greatly exceed this level. Follow on formulae generally have higher concentrations of protein than infant formulae and are therefore not suitable to be given to very young infants. They are permitted by regulation to be sold as suitable for use from the age of 4 months but in clinical practice in this country follow on milks are not introduced before the age of about 6 months.

9.4 Cow's milk

9.4.1 Milks are species specific and they provide a sole source of nutrition for the specific newborn mammal. Humans have used cow's, sheep's and goat's milks to feed their infants and, although these milks contain all essential nutrients, the concentrations of several differ from those in human milk. Whole cow's milk, compared with human milk, contains more protein, less carbohydrate, more riboflavin, less vitamin C and more sodium, potassium, calcium, and magnesium and less iron and copper (Table 9.1). Apart from an increased concentration of total protein in cow's milk, the nature of the proteins is different; casein is the dominant protein in cow's milk and there are higher levels of immunoglobulin G than in human milk. Cow's milk proteins are more allergenic to the human infant than human milk proteins (para 11.1). The small amount of iron in cow's milk is largely present as insoluble phosphate or it is attached to casein in an unabsorbable complex (para 7.3); it is therefore poorly absorbed especially when compared with the iron absorption from human milk.

9.4.2 Because of these and other compositional differences between cow's milk and human milk, unmodified cow's milk has not been recommended in the first 6 months of life for the past 20 years[1]. More recent recommendations have stressed the advantages of continuing breast milk or infant formula as the main drink for the first year particularly to ensure a good intake of iron[2,3]. There have been specific recommendations from individuals in this country and in the USA that whole cow's milk should not be introduced before the age of 12 months and the American Academy of Paediatrics have recently made the same recommendation[151,152,153]. The Working Group recommends that unmodified cow's milk be given as a main drink only after the age of one year. It may be used in small quantities in the preparation of solid foods in the second half of infancy.

9.4.3   After the first year, pasteurised whole cow's milk makes an important contribution to the diet (para 5.6, 8.1). Cow's milk is a poor source of iron and vitamin D but most young children can ensure adequate amounts from other foods, or through the action of sunlight on skin. Where the diet is restricted, or where the opportunity for skin synthesis of vitamin D is limited, feeding with infant formula or follow-on formula should continue (para 11.2) as should vitamin supplements (para 6.6). Western diets rely heavily on cow's milk as a food for children, it provides a substantial proportion of the total intake of protein, calcium and riboflavin. It is therefore important that, as the consumption of milk by the population as a whole declines (Table 8.2), children's diets should be monitored to ensure that they continue to be adequate.

9.4.4   Cow's milk from which the fat has been partly or fully removed is named in relation to a legally enforced fat concentration which must lie between 1.5 to 1.8 per cent by weight for semi-skimmed milk and no more than 0.3 per cent by weight for skimmed milk. As a result energy levels are significantly lower in these milks than in whole cow's milk and fat soluble vitamin levels are also reduced, while potassium and calcium levels are higher (Table 9.2). Semi-skimmed milk is not normally recommended before the age of 2 years, and fully skimmed milk should not be given until the child is over 5 years old (para 5.6).

Table 9.2   *Compositional differences between whole cow's milk, semi-skimmed and fully skimmed milks per 100ml*

		Cow's milk		
		Whole milk	Semi-skimmed	Fully skimmed
Energy	kJ	284	201	144
	kcal	68	47	34
Protein	g	3.3	3.4	3.4
Lactose	g	4.9	5.2	5.2
Fat	g	4.0	1.6	0.1
Vitamin A	ug	57	23	1
Vitamin D	ug	0.03	0.01	Tr
Sodium	mg	57	57	56
Potassium	mg	144	155	155
Calcium	mg	119	124	124
Iron	ug	60	52	62

*   Based on information taken from McCance and Widdowson "The Composition of Foods" 5th edition[44].

9.5 Goat's and sheep's milks

9.5.1   Goat's milk like cow's milk is low in iron, vitamins A and D and is also low in folic acid compared with human and cow's milk. Sheep's milk is also low in iron, vitamin D and folate. It contains 83 µg vitamin A per 100 mls, which is a higher level than in cow's milk (Table 9.1). Although these milks may be perceived as less allergenic or else providing special nourishment, none of these claims have been substantiated[154]. Goat's and sheep's milks should not be given to infants but may be given from the age of one year so long as precautions against mineral and vitamin deficiencies are taken and that due regard is paid to microbiological safety. Specific regulations for goat's and sheep's milk should be in force later in 1994, but until then, these products are controlled by the general provisions of the Food Safety Act 1990.

9.6 Specialised formulae

9.6.1   *Soya infant formulae*   Soya infant formulae are based on soy protein isolate[42]. They may be used from birth and continued beyond the first year if still indicated. Composition is regulated by law in the same way as infant formula based on cow's milk[45] (para 9.2). The 1986 study by MAFF recorded 15 infants (3 per cent of the sample) consuming this product during the survey week[10]. The infant feeding survey of 1990 confirmed that only 2 to 3 per cent of infants were being given soya based infant formulae[9].

9.6.2   These products should not be a first choice unless there is a specific reason for excluding cow's milk products from the diet. They have been developed for infants who are not being breastfed where there is intolerance of cow's milk protein (para 11.1) however, infants at risk of allergy may also become sensitive to soy protein[155], particularly if the cow's milk intolerance has manifested gastrointestinal symptoms. Soya infant formulae are also suitable for bottle fed infants who are lactose intolerant because lactose is replaced by other sugars such as glucose, sucrose and maltose in all brands sold in the UK. Brands which contain no ingredient of animal origin, because carbohydrate is non-lactose and vegetable oils only have been used as the fat source, are acceptable in vegan diets where they provide an important source of nutrients and should be encouraged as the main drink until at least 2 years of age. Absorption of iron, zinc and calcium from these formulae appears to be low, although in practice, weaning diets with soya based infant formulae may be as effective in contributing to an adequate iron status as infant formulae based on cow's milk[156]. Parents should be advised that, because non-milk sugars are included, good weaning practices are particularly important to safeguard dental health; cup feeding should replace bottle feeding after the age of one year and drinks of soya formula between meals or at bedtime are not recommended. Soya drinks, which are not infant formulae, should not be used during weaning. They are deficient in energy and vitamins and calcium content is only 13 mg per 100 mg unless they are fortified[157].

9.6.3   *Infant formulae marketed as less antigenic than standard formulae*
There is long standing clinical experience that foods in which the protein has been modified by hydrolysis are less allergenic than foods using the same

protein whole. Protein may be changed by heating or by enzymatic hydrolysis[158]. Products which contain small molecules are described as "high degree" hydrolysates and include those based on cow's milk or soya proteins as well as hydrolysates of other animal proteins. These products have a distinctive flavour and odour. They are more expensive and they are not generally on open retail sale. They have an important role in the clinical management of highly sensitised individuals with confirmed allergy.

9.6.4   More recently, infant formulae based on cow's milk protein which has undergone "low degree" hydrolysis have been developed[159]. Whole cow's milk protein is modified, but to a lesser extent than "high degree hydrolysis", to offer a product which, it is claimed is less likely to initiate allergic disorders when compared with standard infant formulae. They avoid the distinct flavour and smell of high degree hydrolysate infant formulae. "Low degree" hydrolysate products are intended for infants who, based on their family history, have an increased risk of atopic disease, but who are not yet sensitised. A study in Newfoundland which compared groups of healthy infants at risk fed "low degree" hydrolysate formula, standard cow's milk infant formula and soya infant formula with a group who were exclusively breastfed found that the symptoms of atopic disease were similar in the breastfed and the "low degree" hydrolysate formula up to the age of 18 months and significantly lower than in either of the other two groups[160].

9.7   Drinking water

9.7.1   Public water supplies, whose quality is controlled through legal safeguards[161], are available for almost all of the UK population. Although this water should be safe, all water used to make up infant formula feeds or for giving as a drink of water to infants less than 6 months, should be boiled and cooled. If water for drinking and cooking is taken from the first tap on the mains supply (usually the cold tap in the kitchen) possible problems from deterioration of the water within the domestic plumbing such as microbial contamination or increased lead levels may be avoided. There is now a regime for controlling the quality of private water supplies[162] but, at present, less assurance can be given than for public supplies, particularly in instances such as a shallow well supplying one or two houses. Local Authorities have statutory duties to sample and analyse private water supplies and information on an individual supply may be sought from them.

9.7.2   Bottled waters, other than those labelled "natural mineral water", are expected to conform to essentially the same standards as the public water supply and they are therefore suitable for giving to infants or for preparing feeds. As with tap water, bottled waters should be boiled and cooled before using to make up infant formula feeds. "Natural mineral water" is covered by less comprehensive regulations[163] than tap water and may contain higher concentrations of solutes such as nitrate, sodium, fluoride and sulphate which might lead to solute overload if these waters are given to young infants. The chemical analysis of a natural mineral water is often printed on the label and the manufacturers may provide further information on request. Effervescent water is not suitable for giving to infants.

9.7.3 *Lead* The World Health Organisation has recently advocated a guideline value of 10 micrograms per litre of lead in drinking water[164]. The guideline value may be interpreted as an average over time for an individual and it is not directly comparable to this country's current regulatory limit of 50 micrograms per litre. Limits on lead in water aim to minimise possible long term adverse effects, particularly on neuropsychological development in children. Unacceptable concentrations of lead in water may be found in houses with plumbing systems which contain lead, especially where the water supply is plumbosolvent. Such supplies are typically soft acidic waters, but some hard waters are also able to liberate lead. The extent of the problem has been reduced by the chemical treatment of plumbosolvent waters. In a household where there is still contamination, the concentration of lead in water drawn from a cold tap for consumption, including infant feeding, can usually be reduced substantially by first running a basin full of water to be used for other purposes. Where simple measures fail to reduce the levels of lead concentration in water, lead piping in the house may need to be replaced.

9.7.4 *Other minerals* An excessive intake of sodium is undesirable especially in infancy (para 8.4). Water which has been artificially softened using a salt-regenerated ion exchange water softener or which has been repeatedly boiled should therefore not be used as a drink or for making up infant feeds. High nitrate content of water is one of the causes of methaemoglobinaemia in infants[3]. Where the concentration exceeds 50 milligrams per litre (as nitrate ion) water undertakers are obliged to inform the health authorities and professions in the affected area so as to encourage monitoring for infantile methaemoglobinaemia although this has been detected only very rarely in the United Kingdom. Water with a concentration of nitrate greater than 100 milligrams per litre is not suitable for infant feeding. High concentrations of nitrate and of sulphate occur in some natural mineral waters. High sulphate levels of 400-500 milligrams per litre may be purgative especially in children. Natural mineral waters may contain varying amounts of fluoride and those with high levels and are unsuitable as part of an infant's diet or for making up dried foods or drinks because of the risk of fluorosis of the tooth enamel[165].

9.8 Other drinks

9.8.1 *"Baby" fruit juices and herbal drinks* Recently, manufacturers have developed a range of drinks for infants. "Baby" drinks are available as herbal drinks, fruit juices (ready to feed), and as concentrated juice and dried granulated powder for reconstitution with water. These drinks contain sucrose or glucose or other sugars and most have added vitamin C; they are flavoured with fruit juice or herbal extracts. Baby drinks differ from squashes, juices and soft drinks marketed for adults in having a limited range of additives compatible with those permitted in baby foods (para 10.3). The sugars, which vary in concentration from about 3 g/100 ml in some herbal drinks to about 10 g/100 ml in pure fruit juices, and the acidity can cause caries and erosion of the teeth (para 13.2)[166]. It has also been questioned whether the herbal extracts have pharmacological action although the concentrations may be quite dilute. As with any plant material, certain constituents of herbal extracts can have adverse effects. Manufacturers should ensure that the herbal extracts used do not contain such constituents at doses which could be of concern. The use of herbs which are not commonly consumed as part of the adult diet should be avoided. Further information on the levels of these constituents in herbal drinks would be advisable and on the volumes consumed by babies to allow specific recommendations regarding herbal drinks to be prepared.

9.8.2 *"Soft" drink, colas, squashes* It fruit juices are given other than "baby" fruit juices they should be diluted and offered with meals. If toddlers refuse to eat vitamin C containing foods, vitamin C rich drinks may be used particularly to enhance the absorption of iron from a meal. They should be given from a cup. Other "soft" drinks should not be given during weaning. Colas and several other drinks contain stimulants such as caffeine. Aerated drinks are also quite unsuitable in a weaning diet. Parents may buy "diet" soft drinks to avoid risk to dental health but these drinks are not intended for this age group and if given, infants and young children may have high intakes of artificial sweeteners.

9.8.3 *Tea* Tea is commonly given to pre-school children. Preliminary data from the National Diet and Nutrition Survey (para 2.3) show that during the 4 day recording period, 38 per cent of children aged 1½ to 2½ years drank tea of whom about half sweetened it with sucrose[11]. Tea is not advised as a main drink for infants and young children. Tannin in tea binds with iron and other minerals[167] and reduces their bioavailability (para 7.3) and if sugar is added there is risk to dental health.

9.8.4 Drinks other than breast milk, infant formula and follow on milk contribute little to nutrient needs and if consumed to excess or between meals, they are likely to reduce appetite for more nutrient dense drinks and foods. Cooled boiled water can satisfactorily quench thirst. Fruit juices should be diluted. "Baby drinks" are not needed, but if given they should be used sparingly and then only at meal times and parents should be advised to use a cup to safeguard infant dental health. Sweetened drinks and naturally sweet drinks taken from feeding bottles should be strongly discouraged.

9.9 **What drinks are given to children?** The 1990 Government survey of infant feeding practices found that 37 per cent of infants received infant formula from birth and that by the age of 4 weeks the majority of babies in the UK were being fed exclusively on infant formula. Cow's milk had been introduced as a drink by 3 per cent of mothers by the age of 4/5 months. By 9/10 months, 59 per cent of babies were still being given infant formula or follow on formula and 76 per cent of all mothers were giving their babies liquid cow's milk in some way, a fall from 88 per cent in 1985. It was used as the main "milk" drink by 40 per cent and 17 per cent used it as a second "milk"[9]. The 1986 study of infants aged 6 to 12 months found that cow's milk was being consumed by two-thirds of the group with a trend to increasing consumption by the older infants in the group. The same study found that baby herbal drinks, fruit juices and powdered drinks were being consumed by up to a quarter of the younger members of the group but this rate declined as the infants approached one year of age. Fruit squashes were increasingly used as the child approached a year. Water was infrequently used. By 11/12 months of age 13 per cent of mothers reported giving tea to their infants and this rate increases with age (para 9.8)[10].

10. Solids foods given in the weaning diet

The Working Group recommends that

- non-wheat cereals and pureed fruit, vegetables and potatoes are suitable first weaning foods. Salt should not be added and additional sugars should be limited to that needed for palatability of sour fruits. Between six and nine months of age the amount and variety of foods including meat, fish, eggs, all cereals and pulses should be increased and the number of "milk" feeds reduced. Food consistency should progress from pureed through minced/mashed to finely chopped. By the age of one year the diet should be mixed and varied (para 10.1);

- in the later stages of weaning, three meals per day are suggested with two or three snacks in addition (para 10.1.4);

- the labels of commercial baby foods should provide consistent information which is understandable to parents (para 10.3.3);

- foods given during weaning should be prepared, handled and stored in a hygienic way (para 10.5).

10.1 Introducing solids

10.1.1 Weaning foods have traditionally been staged in relation to age and development and while this is helpful, it is only a general indicator. Infants vary in the rates at which they develop feeding skills and habits and often they do not match the stages, for instance, where solids are not offered until 5 or 6 months and the infant begins first by putting pieces of food into the mouth. An example of practical dietetic guidance for this age is provided in Annex III.

10.1.2 *Initial stage: 4 to 6 months*   In the initial stage of weaning the aim is to accustom the infant to take food from a spoon. The first foods offered are of smooth consistency and bland taste. This contribution of non-milk foods to the energy and nutrient intakes is small, and breast milk or infant formula continue to provide the main nutrition. Suitable first foods are cereal such as infant baby rice or pureed home-cooked rice, mashed potato, custard, plain (unsweetened) yoghurt and pureed non-fibrous vegetables. When the infant has accepted eating from a spoon, different tastes and textures can be introduced. Well cooked pureed meat, pulses, fruit and a wider variety of cereals will offer new experiences. There is individual variation in the duration of the initial stage of weaning which may last a short time or may extend for several weeks.

10.1.3 *Second stage: 6 to 9 months* Once a variety of food is accepted from a spoon two to three times daily, the infant is ready for the second stage. Solid foods begin to be important providers of energy and nutrients as the infant becomes less dependent on milk. In the second stage of weaning the infant experiences different textures of food and stronger tastes. The infant will usually begin to put foods into the mouth. This can be encouraged by giving soft finger foods such as toast, cooked green beans, and carrots and soft raw fruits such as banana and pear. At this stage these foods will be more sucked than bitten and chewed. Family foods can be mashed or blended to a texture containing some soft lumps (eg mashed banana); vegetables need to be cooked until soft and meats will still need to be coarsely pureed. Commercial infant foods should be "second stage" type. The taste of food can be less plain; adding salt or sugars is not recommended.

10.1.4 *Third stage: 9 to 12+ months* This stage of weaning marks progression to the more mature diet of three main meals interspersed with snacks and/or drinks of milk in addition. Cooked vegetables need only be chopped and some salad vegetables can be included. Meat may need to be minced or finely chopped. Finger foods are popular at this age and are a preliminary to full self-feeding. Small cubes of fruits, vegetables, potato, toast, cheese or soft meat should be included at each meal so that the infant is encouraged to participate in self-feeding. By the end of the third stage separately prepared foods are no longer needed and the full family diet can be offered (para 10.2.2) .

10.1.5 Several different foods and drinks from all of the food groups should be offered to ensure an adequate intake of all nutrients (see Annex III). Most infants are given both home prepared and commercial foods as the diet is diversified. Diets during weaning should aim to provide RNI levels of nutrients, but intakes should be assessed over a period of time. Weaning diets with a proportion of fortified commercial foods may more readily approach RNI values especially for minerals although the bioavailability of added minerals such as iron may be low (para 7.3).

10.2 Family Foods

10.2.1 A weaning diet of home prepared foods provides an excellent start to mixed feeding. A wide range of basic household food can be used, (with the exception of foods commonly thought to be allergenic during the early weeks (para 11.1) and foods excluded on food safety grounds (para 10.5)) provided it has been rendered to a satisfactory texture. The nutrient content of home prepared foods reflects that of the foods used. Data on the nutrient composition of home prepared weaning foods are scarce. Recent analyses found that the nutrient content of home prepared weaning foods were very variable but there was a tendency for the foods sampled to be low in fat, protein and iron; many had low energy densities which was ascribed to lower mean sugars contents when compared with manufactured foods[168]. Home prepared pureed foods can be supplemented with cereal foods and snacks and a diversity of peeled and cut up fresh fruit while breast milk, infant formula and, later, follow-on formula and cow's milk remain significant providers of energy and nutrients.

10.2.2   Most foods need to be softened by cooking and then pureed, mashed or chopped. Young infants accept bland tasting food and it should contain no additional salt and only a minimum of sugars for sour fruits. Once the infant is more used to a diversity of tastes, prepared dishes such as cauliflower cheese, or beef, sprouts and potatoes, or peaches and custard can be rendered to the correct consistency. For infants fully integrated into family meals, food can be prepared without added salt or sugars for the whole family, a portion reserved for the infant's meal, and the remainder of the family can then add flavourings such as salt or spices to their own taste. When food is made into a puree or mashed, some water may need to be added but not so that the food is sloppy and diluted. Meat can be pureed satisfactorily in this way. Preparing foods as a puree or chopped dish for infants is sometimes very easy but it can also be messy and the food may have an unattractive colour. On the other hand, many parents like to know exactly what ingredients have been used to prepare food for their baby.

10.3.   Commercial baby foods

10.3.1   Commercial baby foods are intended to contribute to a mixed weaning diet of family foods and commercial products. The manufacturers provide products which reflect family eating patterns, some are intended to provide whole courses and others, such as pureed vegetables or minced meat, provide one constituent of a meal to be combined with other commercial or home prepared foods.

10.3.2   *Ready to eat "wet" foods*   in cans and jars are prepared by a standard procedure of recipe formulation, preparation, cooking, chopping and retorting at temperatures and conditions which vary with the type of product. *Dried baby foods* are prepared according to defined recipes. The food is then passed through a roller drier which, in a matter of seconds, cooks and dries the food. The baby's feed is then prepared in the home by adding either water or "milk" as stated in the instructions on the packet, "milk" which may be breast milk, infant formula and after six months, cow's milk or follow-on formula will result in a more nutrient dense feed than if water is used. *Cereal based weaning foods* are processed in various ways. Pre-cooked cereals may be used and these require no further cooking before use. Enzyme-treated cereals are prepared by allowing enzymes to transform the starch into dextrin, maltodextrin, maltose and/or dextrose. Rusks and biscuits are prepared by baking and may be used directly or crumbled into milk or water. Biscuits consist of cereals with added whole milk protein or other milk components. Most rusks and biscuits contain sugars as well as cereal products and only some are gluten free.

10.3.3   Commercial products are labelled with instructions about use, the ingredients and nutritional information which is often based on what portion of the daily RNI the product contributes. Other information is given, for instance if the food is totally meat free and suitable for vegetarians or if it is gluten free. There are also concerns, in order to protect dental health, that information about sugars content of manufactured foods and drinks used in the weaning diet should be given on labels. There are no commercial baby foods which use halal or kosher food preparation methods and this may result in an unduly restricted diet. If such products become available they will need to be appropriately labelled (para 11.2). Manufacturers should ensure that the information is clearly presented and understandable to the purchaser.

10.3.4 The Codex Alimentarius Commission, which is jointly sponsored by the World Health Organisation and the Food and Agricultural Organisation of the United Nations, has set compositional standards for baby foods[169]. More recently, the European Community Scientific Committee for Food prepared an expert report on the Essential Requirements for Weaning Foods[170] and the European Commission has now issued a draft Directive on processed cereal-based foods and baby foods for infants and young children based on the report's recommendations[171]. It deals with the foods used as raw ingredients, energy and nutrient compositions and package labelling. Regulations governing weaning foods need to take account of the diversity of use of individual commercial products and the varying contributions they make to the diet as a whole.

10.3.5 *Additives in baby foods* The UK Government published an expert report on additives in food specially prepared for infants and young children from the Food Advisory Committee on Toxicity of Chemicals in Food, Consumer Products and the Environment[172]. This recommended that additives should only be used where there is strong justification on technological grounds; they should be kept to a minimum whilst allowing the current range of products to continue to be manufactured. The report also considered the safety of individual additives used in foods specially prepared for infants and young children and whether it is acceptable to add flavourings to commercial weaning foods. The Food Advisory Committee recognised the potential benefits of weaning foods which have flavour, and possible consequences of providing infants and young children with a very bland diet. However, it did not consider that these factors substantiated a case of need for flavourings other than the flavoured constituents of a normal diet. Nonetheless, it was recognised that it is not always practicable to use only foodstuffs for flavouring. The report recommended that manufacturers should use only natural food substances, such as fruits, wherever possible, to flavour foods specially prepared for infants. Where this was not possible, only extracts and/or essential oils from foods, herbs and spices which are commonly consumed as part of the UK diet should be used at levels which do not result in intakes exceeding that from consumption of a normal diet. Manufacturers were asked to note the limits for certain undesirable substances present in natural flavourings, as specified in the Flavourings in Food Regulations 1992[173]. The Food Advisory Committee did not consider there was a case of need for nature-identical or artificial flavouring substances so did not recommend their use.

10.3.6   The European Commission's Scientific Committee for Food has also given advice on additives in foods specially prepared for infants and young children[170]. A Council Directive on food additives other than colours and sweeteners[174], which includes an annex covering additives in foods specially prepared for infants and young children, has recently been agreed.

10.4   Choice of foods

10.4.1   Mothers in the UK tend to choose commercial baby foods such as baby rice, rusks and other cereal products as first foods and sometimes first stage vegetables or fruits[9,10]. The practice of first introducing a small amount of unsalted unsweetened home prepared and pureed fruit or vegetable is strongly encouraged[175] but this start to weaning has had limited popularity. Preparing home made foods needs shopping and cooking skills and some mothers may not feel confident that they know which foods are most suitable. If parents are giving predominantly manufactured foods, it is important that home prepared foods should also be given to accustom the infant to the greater ranges of flavour and texture that they provide. An infant who has been given a diet of commercial foods may later be reluctant to change to home prepared food.

10.4.2   Parents need to balance apparent extra costs of commercial foods against the time saving and convenience of these foods especially in the first stages of weaning when only small amounts are used. Once the volume of food eaten increases, cost probably has a greater influence on the choice of diet. By 9 months of age infants should readily consume a bowlful of mashed family foods and parents gain in confidence that their baby is growing and developing normally and is enjoying the food that is prepared at home. The use of commercial baby foods declines rapidly in the second year. The National Diet and Nutrition Survey of pre-school children recorded only 4 per cent of children aged 1½ to 2½ years who ate any such foods over a 4 day period of dietary recording[11].

10.5   Food hygiene

10.5.1   Many foods can carry micro-organisms which cause foodborne illness. If food is not properly handled, cooked or stored, it can provide a suitable environment for the multiplication of bacteria. Babies and young children are more at risk of severe illness from food borne infection than older children or adults.

10.5.2   Home prepared food should start with fresh or canned foods, or chilled or frozen foods which are within the manufacturer's recommended "use-by" date. The utensils and appliances must be as clean as possible and both parent and child should start with clean hands. Not all frozen foods need to be defrosted before cooking, many should not be. The food needs to be cooked thoroughly, and, if it is a re-heated meal, the heating must be thorough. However, care must be taken to ensure that the food is not so hot when it is given to eat that the mouth is scalded. This is especially important when food has been heated in a microwave oven which results in very high temperature at the centre of the food mass; a short cooling period with a stir of the food is recommended. Partly eaten food should be thrown away. Prepared food which is being kept for a short period in the refrigerator should be wrapped or covered, to reduce the chance of coming into contact with raw food. Parents may wish to freeze small portions of home prepared food. This should be done as soon as the food has cooled after cooking and not after a long delay when bacteria may already have multiplied in the food. If egg is given during weaning it must be cooked until the white and yolk are solid[176].

10.5.3   Commercial foods are required by food law to be safe up to the point of sale. However, the handling and storage of packaged food before and after it has been opened may make commercially produced food as vulnerable to contamination as home produced foods. Cooking times and temperatures in recipes or on labels should be followed. This is also relevant to using microwave ovens. If an infant leaves food on the plate this should be thrown away and part-used tins and jars of commercial foods should also be discarded.

11. Special considerations

11.1 Food intolerance, allergy and anaphylaxis

The Working Group recommends that

- where there is a family history of atopy or gluten enteropathy, mothers should be encouraged to breastfeed for six months or longer. Weaning before four months should particularly be discouraged and the introduction of foods traditionally regarded as allergenic should be delayed until six months at the earliest (para 11.1.4);

- there should be further investigation of dietary factors which initiate atopic disorders (para 11.1.6).

11.1.1   Food intolerance covers any non-psychological undesirable reaction to a specific food or ingredient; there is a variable aetiology[177]. The reaction may be toxic, idiosyncratic, metabolic, or allergic.

11.1.2   *Food allergy*   Allergy is a clinical syndrome of hypersensitivity which is immunologically mediated. A humoral mechanism which relies on specific antibodies such as IgE, IgG or IgA can be involved and/or cell mediated immunity through T-lymphocytes and macrophages. Genetic factors, among others, are known to determine the risk of allergy. The risk of a child developing an allergic disorder more than doubles if there is a family history of parent or sibling with atopic disease[178]. Food allergy can cause, or contribute to, a variety of conditions including eczema, urticaria, hay fever, bronchial asthma and gastrointestinal disorders, especially diarrhoea with failure to thrive. Food antigens which have commonly been implicated include cow's milk protein, eggs, nuts, wheat and shellfish (para 3.3).

11.1.3   *Food induced anaphylaxis*   Infants or children can, very rarely, have a severe allergic reaction on the first occasion a food is consumed. The signs are a rapid onset of red itchy weals and oedema with circulatory collapse which may be life threatening. The reaction is presumed to be a response to a food to which the individual was sensitised in utero or during breastfeeding through mother to child transmission of the antigen. After the first episode it is important to identify the allergen and exclude it from the diet[179]. Re-introduction of the allergen to the diet after a few years should only be attempted under expert clinical supervision.

11.1.4   *Management of food allergy*   Infants are most vulnerable to the initiation of food allergy in the first months of life (para 3.3). Where there is a family history of atopic disease exclusive breastfeeding should particularly be encouraged for 4 to 6 months and preferably longer. The preventive effect of breastfeeding is further enhanced if the mother's diet during lactation excludes common allergens[180]. An early start to weaning should be discouraged and allergenic foods should not be included in the diet until 6 months of age. It is no longer recommended that all infants be introduced to new foods one at a time but is probably still advisable where there is a strong family history of allergy. It is important when advising parents about how to avoid allergy, that simple measures such as reducing contact with non-food allergens by avoiding smoking and keeping children away from pets should also be included[181].

11.1.5 For the infant who is already highly sensitised to whole cow's milk protein, semi-elemental diets which incorporate "high degree" hydrolysates of cow's milk protein or other protein sources make an essential contribution but they are only indicated exceptionally under clinical supervision (para 9.6). Infants with established sensitisation to cow's milk protein should not be given "low degree" hydrolysates because of their increased risk of anaphylactic reactions. To prevent the development of allergy, where there is a family history of intolerance to cow's milk protein, "low degree" whey protein hydrolysates have been used in several countries although there is no experience in the UK[159] (para 9.6).

11.1.6 Infant formulae based on soy protein isolate (para 9.6) have been used for infants who are not being breastfed where there is increased risk or established intolerance of cow's milk protein (para 9.6). Soya is itself allergenic. However, older infants given soya infant formula because of the development of allergy to cow's milk protein may tolerate soya because they have already grown beyond the age of greatest risk of sensitisation. As weaning progresses, soya infant formula may continue to be given as the milk drink from a cup for as long as it is accepted.

11.1.7 If any substantial degree of dietary manipulation is needed the advice of a paediatric dietitian should be obtained. If the range of foods in the diet is reduced during weaning, nutrient deficiencies become more likely. The management of allergies in young children is demanding on parents and on professional advisers. The proportion of young children affected by allergies appears to be increasing although the extent to which food allergies are responsible is unclear and there should be further investigation of the dietary factors which initiate atopic disorders.

11.1.8 *Coeliac Disease* Coeliac disease is associated with damage to the small intestinal mucosa which leads to malabsorption of nutrients. The mechanism has not been fully clarified nor is the exact epitope(s) concerned fully identified although prolamins from wheat, rye, barley and oats have been implicated. To prevent coeliac disease the cereals given to infants less than six months should preferably be gluten free, such as rice or maize. Coeliac disease is treated by excluding gluten from the diet.

11.1.9 The genetic basis of the susceptibility to coeliac disease is unknown and it is not possible to predict the individuals who will be affected. Coeliac disease commonly manifests in the weaning period when a diverse diet which includes foods containing gluten is first encountered. The prevalence of the disease in European countries is about 1 in 1000. Prevalence varies over time[20] and between countries[182]. Gluten sensitive infants who are breastfed and who are introduced to gluten relatively late may not present clinically during weaning, although the disorder manifests at an older age and the cumulative prevalence of coeliac disease is unaffected. This delay in clinical presentation is valuable because nutrition and health are spared from adverse effects during the vulnerable early years of rapid growth.

11.2 Influences of culture, religion and ethnicity on the weaning diet

The Working Group recommends that

● **infants being weaned on diets restricted in animal protein should particularly be offered a variety of foods at each meal. Protein sources should be mixed. Each meal should provide vitamin C, and an energy supplement from a fat source should be considered if there are doubts about the adequacy of energy intake (para 11.2.4);**

● **the range of commercial weaning foods should be enlarged to offer a wider choice to those with special cultural or religious dietary requirements and they should be appropriately labelled (para 11.2.7).**

11.2.1   Dietary practices are powerfully influenced by culture and by religious beliefs, common patterns adhered to by minority groups in this country are listed in Annex IV. In the UK, as elsewhere, ethnic minority communities often wish to retain patterns of life which they have brought to this country and which differ from local traditions. New foods, different ways of preparing food and a wider range of tastes have enriched the British diet. However, there are difficulties for some ethnic groups and these may adversely effect the nutrition of infants and young children during weaning. New mothers may be isolated and deprived of support from their wider community network of family, friends and informal advisors. They may not speak English and they may not know how to get advice. The foods on sale may be unfamiliar and known foods may be difficult to find. Their opportunities for choice and experimentation may be further restricted by low income (para 14.3). These difficulties are greater for new immigrants.

11.2.2   Low rates of breastfeeding in immigrant communities tend to match low rates across populations in inner city areas. In 1974-6, of infants living in Glasgow, 48 per cent of Nigerian origin, 21 per cent of Asian (mainly Punjabi) origin and 2 per cent of Hong Kong origin were breastfed[183]. This contrasts with rates of breastfeeding in the countries of origin which exceeded 80 per cent in all cases. At the same time, the breastfeeding rates of indigenous Scottish infants in Glasgow was only one per cent and this pattern of virtually exclusive artificial feeding probably influenced new arrivals from other countries not to breastfeed. More recent surveys have also shown low rates of breastfeeding in Pakistani Asians in Bradford[184], in Asians from the northern subcontinent in Leeds[185] (Annex I) and in Bangladeshis in London[186], but, except for the Leeds study, breastfeeding rates were similarly low among local white mothers. The ages at which solids are first given tend to reflect the patterns for the whole population in inner city areas, although there are variations between studies[183,187,185].

11.2.3 During weaning, some infants from Asian and Chinese minority groups receive large amounts of infant formula or cow's milk as their main source of nutrition for an inappropriately long time. These drinks cannot provide adequately for nutrient and energy needs beyond about 6 months, and there is risk of iron and other micronutrient deficiencies especially when cow's milk dominates the diet during infancy (para 9.4)[188,189,184]. Two practices which are more common in Asian communities are prolonged bottle feeding and adding sugar or honey to drinks. More than 90 per cent of Asian infants were using a feeding bottle over the age of 2 years in the Leeds study[185]. Sweetened drinks given in bottles predispose to dental caries (para 13.2). While Asian mothers acknowledged the relationship between eating "sweets" and dental decay, the adverse effect on the teeth of bottle feeding sweetened drinks was not recognised[190]. Prolonged bottle feeding without experiencing the variety of taste and texture of solid weaning foods can lead to rejection of the mixed diet by the young child later. In communities where bottle feeding is known to be practised into the second year education should be directed at learning to drink from a cup and encouraging earlier diversity and solid foods in the diet.

11.2.4 *Vegetarian diets* (see Annex IV for definitions) Hindu parents are particularly likely to give a vegetarian diet, as do a proportion of parents from all cultures. They may choose to do so because of their religion or on a basis of personal belief. Less restrictive lactovegetarian or lactovovegetarian diets can be fully satisfactory during weaning although parents may need to be educated about how best to meet their child's nutritional needs (para 14.3). Such diets tend to be low in energy and bulky and children may not manage to consume large amounts. Where there are doubts about the adequacy of energy intakes, a supplement from a fat source should be considered although this should only be done with care to avoid a lower protein to energy ratio in the diet. High levels of phytate and other inhibitors in some foods may reduce the bioavailability of the dietary minerals especially iron, zinc and copper (para 5.5). It is important for vegetarian diets to contain high levels of vitamin C because this enhances the absorption of these micronutrients (para 6.2).

11.2.5 *Vegan diet* British breastfed children born to vegan mothers and weaned on a vegan diet are reported to grow and develop normally. However, the diets of vegan children tend to contain less energy than those of non vegetarian children and these children tend to be smaller and lighter than standards for the general population[191]. Care is required in choice of plant foods for example in order that amino acids can be complemented adequately and that sufficient fat is included. Fruits and vegetables tend to be more bulky than cereals and large amounts can lead to a reduced energy density of the diet. High levels of phytate and other mineral inhibitors are also found in seeds, bran products and some legumes. A vegan diet strictly adhered to cannot provide vitamin B12, and riboflavin intakes are also grossly inadequate. B12 stores in the newborn and breast fed infants of vegans may relate more to the dietary ingestion of the vitamin by the mother than to maternal body stores[192]. Vitamin B12 is recycled into the gut and this may result in a long period before depletion. Vegans accept the need for dietary supplementation which includes riboflavin and vitamin B12 (para 6.2).

11.2.6 *Macrobiotic, Rastafarian and other very restricted diets* Children fed very restricted macrobiotic types of diet are particularly at risk and there are a number of reports of malnutrition in infants fed macrobiotic, Rastafarian and other vegan like diets. There have been severe problems including deaths from energy and protein malnutrition, as well as iron, vitamin B12[193], calcium, zinc and vitamin D deficiencies for example in infants fed cereal gruels with a grossly inadequate energy and protein content. These diets cannot be recommended[194,195,38,196].

11.2.7 In some religions meat should not be consumed unless it has been slaughtered ritually. For Jews, meat that is not kosher, and for Muslims meat that is not halal, is unclean. Parents who cannot find acceptable meat to cook in the home, or who cannot prepare it, nor find acceptable manufactured foods, may resort to a meat free diet. Occasionally the diet becomes restricted to cow's milk and manufactured baby desserts with resulting nutritional deficiency and a higher risk of dental caries (para 13.2). Mothers need support from their community and from health professionals (para 14.3) to help provide adequate and diverse diets during weaning. Fathers and male household members should also be involved since they are frequently the main purchasers of foods for their families. Food manufacturers should enlarge their ranges to meet the needs of those who wish to choose commercial products and labelling should give enough information to allow foods to be distinguished according to religious requirements.

11.2.8 Vitamin D is naturally present in only a limited range of foods which includes oily fish and to a smaller extent, eggs and possibly also meat (para 6.3). A major source of vitamin D is through synthesis in the skin. Asian children are particularly at risk of vitamin D deficiency (para 6.3) as they may be subject to dietary restrictions or their culture and environment may not provide opportunities to expose their skin to summer sunlight. Skin pigmentation causes lower rates of vitamin D synthesis. Children from ethnic minorities who are thought to be at risk should particularly be encouraged to take vitamin supplements to age 5 years or longer (para 6.6).

11.2.9 Changes in patterns of life and eating habits have occurred, particularly in the second generation, and it is important that education for ethnic minority groups is based on a knowledge of current dietary practices. A survey of infant feeding and weaning practices and of growth rates of babies from Gujarati, Punjabi, Pakistani and Bangladeshi communities as well as a group of white mothers resident in the same locality has recently been commissioned by the Department of Health. Fieldwork begins in autumn 1994 and the newborn infants will be followed up for the first 15 months of life. A published report is expected in 1997.

11.3 Weaning infants who were born pre-term.

11.3.1 Advising when to begin weaning a baby born pre-term may present difficulties. If weaning begins at an equivalent age of 4 months post term, breast milk or infant formula provide the only source of nourishment for very many months and parents become impatient for change. Most infants mature in response to external stimuli and may appear to be ready for more diversity than milk alone offers. A reasonable compromise may need to be adopted such that weaning can be advised when the infant weighs at least 5 kg, has lost the extrusion reflex and is able to eat from a spoon.

11.3.2 Infants born pre-term are nutritionally vulnerable. They have reduced stores of iron (para 7.3) and also probably zinc (para 8.7)[197] which become exhausted more quickly than the larger stores in liver and haemoglobin in term infants. Bone mineralisation is also commonly poor[198]. It is important that the diet ensures adequate sources of energy and nutrients in forms which can be absorbed readily by the infant. Breast milk exerts a favourable effect on neurodevelopment of infants born pre-term[65]. Special infant formulae are also available for feeding to newborn pre-term infants. When solids are introduced and throughout the process of weaning, particular attention is needed to ensure that the dietary intake fully meets energy and nutrient needs[199]. Fussy eaters who are difficult to feed may need expert advice from a paediatric dietitian to ensure that the diet remains adequate at all times.

12. The influence of the weaning diet on growth and health

12.1 Failure to thrive

The Working Group recommends that

- **infants and young children who are failing to thrive should be identified as early as possible, and a nutritional cause should be investigated (para 12.1.3);**

- **there should be further research into nutritional causes of failure to thrive (para 12.1.6).**

12.1.1 Growth in infancy is usually assessed by serial recordings of weight. Infant length and head circumference may be used in addition, but it is difficult to measure length accurately for routine surveillance. Inadequate growth may first be suspected when successive measurements cross reference centile values with a downward trend. Infants and young children who do not grow in accordance with expectations based on population norms, are described as failing to thrive. Reference standards for these measurements were set out as charts by Tanner in 1966[200,201]. New growth charts which draw on several UK data sets are now being prepared.

12.1.2 Several definitions have been used for failure to thrive, for instance, a downward deviation of weight gain during the first year from a birth weight which was above the 3rd population centile on conventional growth standards, to weights lying persistently below that centile for at least 3 months[202]. However this definition does not include the child who, although relatively large for age is failing to grow in weight or length with the expected increments but where values do not fall below the lower third centile. A refinement to this definition is that baseline weight is taken between 4 to 8 weeks after birth when an infant born "light-for-dates", because of maternal factors, might be expected to have caught up weight expected on the basis of genetic potential[203]. Even so, some infants, born small for dates, have not gained weight fully by eight weeks of age. Identifying inadequate growth in the first 2 years of life is further complicated because breastfed infants and infants fed infant formula exhibit slightly different growth patterns (para 5.1).

12.1.3 The first sign of failure to thrive is a declining rate of weight gain, later the rate of gain in length becomes less than expected and the rate of gain in head circumference also declines. Cognitive deficit is a feature of more severe and prolonged failure to thrive and this is particularly seen in developing countries[204]. Several clinical conditions may be associated with failure to thrive including neurological, gastro-intestinal and cardiac diseases[205]. Where no such disorder can be implicated the term non-organic failure to thrive has been used and feeding problems or difficulties in child-parent interaction may be causal, or the child may be suffering neglect or abuse. To avoid risk of adverse consequences, failure to thrive should be diagnosed and treated without delay.

12.1.4   The prevalence of non-organic failure to thrive in a cohort of inner city newborn children from South London who were monitored for 4 years, was 3.5 per cent. There were differences according to ethnic group; no children from the African child population, but 15 per cent of Asian children from the Indian subcontinent, were affected[206]. Only 20 per cent of children diagnosed as failing to thrive by this observational research study were found retrospectively to have been referred by the community or primary health care services for expert advice.

12.1.5   Distinguishing between "organic" and "non-organic" failure to thrive may not be helpful. Social, clinical and psychological factors may all be contributing to cause a child to fail to thrive. Several dietary and nutritional factors have been implicated in the development of this condition. Energy and nutrient intakes may be inadequate because of inappropriate diets, due, for instance, to prolonged reliance on milk alone (para 11.2) or because the diet contains too much bulky low energy food (para 5.5). In other circumstances young children may consume snacks and large volumes of dilute juices which reduce the appetite for more nutrient dense foods. The nutrient intake may not provide for increased requirements associated with infections[207] and these children frequently have poor appetites as do children with iron deficiency (para 7.2). Clinical disorders, may reduce the absorption of food.

12.1.6   Feeding and behavioural problems may be significant determinants of a child's failure to thrive. The child may show no signs of being hungry, nor is there apparent eagerness to feed when food is offered[206]. In other cases the child may show determination not to accept new tastes or textures which can result in a restricted diet inappropriate for the child's age. Sometimes infants and young children are not willing to sit down and concentrate on eating or they may be very slow eaters with apparent difficulties in eating and swallowing so that meal times are very prolonged. These difficulties reflect extreme examples of behaviour patterns common to most young children at some stage. Mothers and other carers differ in their skills in overcoming these eating problems. If the mother is not very interested in her child or is indifferent to food, or is repelled by messy food, or if she is determined to establish control of the child's eating patterns with resulting conflict, the outcome is likely to be that less food is consumed. She may be depressed with puerperal psychosis although this does not necessarily mean that her parenting skills are inadequate[208]. Further investigations of the nutritional causes which contribute to failure to thrive should help to improve the dietary and behavioural advice that can be offered to these children and their parents.

12.1.7   Where several factors have combined to make feeding difficult, the mother, or other carer, may benefit from time spent regularly with the baby in a specially equipped and staffed day centre. Sustained contact with other mothers and with professional experts may reveal unsatisfactory feeding relationships and habits and mothers can be helped to regain their confidence and increase their understanding about how to feed their babies more satisfactorily[209] (para 14.3).

12.2 Body fatness

The Working Group recommends that

● **criteria for defining fatness in young children should be standardised (para 12.2.2). The determinants of fatness in young children, its prevalence and population changes in degrees of fatness should be examined and short and long-term consequences assessed (para 12.2.3).**

12.2.1 The average fat mass trebles between birth and 4 months of age and by 6 months infants are commonly chubby and fat contributes a quarter of body weight. There is probably a physiological change at this age with a gradual decline in fatness[210] as proportionately more lean than fat tissue is deposited. Fat laid down in the first 6 months after birth provides an important store for use at times of low energy intake during weaning when eating behaviour may be capricious or when there are increased energy demands due, for instance, to infections.

12.2.2 There are no agreed criteria to assess relative fatness in children. In population studies the measure most commonly used for adults, weight/height^2, shows an increase in the first year, then a decrease in both sexes to the age of 6 years when a second increase follows. The coefficient of variation of this ratio in the population under 3 years of age is small[211]. Skinfold thickness measurements do not assess internal fat deposits and the standard regression equations, which allow a measure of total body fatness from skinfold measurements for adults are not appropriate for this age. Criteria to define relative fatness, including overweight and underweight, should be standardised so that prevalence studies and population changes can be evaluated.

12.2.3 Obesity in adults increases the risk of chronic disease and it is therefore important to know whether fatness in toddlers predicts obesity, or other measures of risk in adult life[212] and whether dietary modification in childhood might prevent adult obesity. However, the relationship between fatness as a child and adult obesity is not clear[213]. Most fat infants do not become obese adults although a large proportion of obese adults were fat infants. Twin studies have shown that there is a genetic component to the tendency to obesity although this is only one of several risk factors[214]. There should be further research into the natural history of obesity including an assessment of the short and long term consequences of fatness in infancy and early childhood.

12.2.4   Feeding practices which may contribute to fatness during weaning include continued use of bottle feeding with large amounts of formula or cow's milk *in addition to* an adequate weaning diet. Lower levels of energy expenditure have been associated with higher degrees of body fatness in under-fives[215,216]. All toddlers need exercise, if possible outside the home and they should be encouraged to walk instead of sitting in pushchairs. Children should do things for themselves such as undressing or dressing and feeding themselves. Many hours spent viewing television reduces activity levels and, in some families predisposes to snacking – both factors which may contribute to the development of obesity. Very fat toddlers with obese parents are at the highest risk of persisting obesity and their parents should be given special advice to avoid overfeeding their young children and to encourage them to provide opportunities for regular physical activity.

12.3   Early nutrition and adult health

The Working Group recommends that

● **priority should be given to continuing investigations into the effect of diet and nutrition of the infant and young child on health in childhood and adult life (para 12.3.5).**

12.3.1   There has been long-standing interest in the extent to which adult health may be determined by factors in early life[217]. Recent epidemiological studies have identified factors reflecting nutritional status in foetal life and infancy, including birth weight and infant growth rate, which appear also to be linked with adult health[55]. However, genetic endowment as well as factors such as social and economic circumstances also affect correlations between health and nutritional status in early and in later life[218], and the relative importance of several risk factors in modifying health and disease in infancy and childhood or, independently, in later life, remains unclear[219].

12.3.2   Prospective studies are more likely to provide definitive data. The British longitudinal study of children born in 1970 found an inverse relationship between birth weight and systolic blood pressure at age 10 years (9,921 subjects)[220]. On the other hand, a longitudinal study of 758 infants born preterm found no relationship between fetal nutrition or early growth after delivery and the level of blood pressure at aged $7\frac{1}{2}$ to 8 years[221]. The Medical Research Council National Study of Health and Development has followed up over 3,000 adults since birth in 1946. In this group lower birth weight, body shape and the father's blood pressure were the best predictors of higher blood pressure in adult life[220]. Results from this study will be particularly informative as the survivors grow older and chronic disease more prevalent. In the USA, the Bogalusa longitudinal study from infancy, has provided extensive and valuable data about the significance of early influences on the development of disease[222]. However, because of life style difference between this country and Southern USA, the relevance of the observations from Bogalusa to the population of the United Kingdom must be interpreted cautiously.

12.3.3 Alternatively disease in adult populations can be compared retrospectively with health and nutritional status in early life. Thus, rates of ischemic heart disease[223] and stroke, and the associated conditions hypertension and non-insulin dependent diabetes in groups of middle aged and older men correlated closely with lower rates of growth and development during fetal life and infancy[224,225,226]. Groups of adults who had lower levels of plasma fibrinogen and blood clotting factor VII tended to come from groups with higher body weights at one year[227]. These studies, most of which have been limited to males, suggest that groups with high rates of growth during fetal and infant life are at lower risk of certain diseases in late middle age.

12.3.4 Nutritional status in early life could be a factor in determining these relationships. Apart from influencing birth weight and infant health and growth, nutritional status may also influence "programming" of organs during development, and there may be but a short time span during which this process must be completed if an organ is to mature fully. Periods of nutritional inadequacy might prevent the development of new blood vessels needed to allow specific body organs and tissues to develop to their full potential. This mechanism could explain the relationship between low birth weight and diabetes if nutrient deficiency during fetal life, apart from causing poor foetal growth, also were to prevent the pancreatic beta cells multiplying and maturing. The infant would then be born with a permanent deficit of pancreatic beta cells which condition predisposed to diabetes. Alternatively, damage to the immune processes in early life may be permanent which may provide another possible explanation for the predisposition to diabetes in later life of individuals who were born small. These and other plausible biological mechanisms have suggested factors related to nutritional status which could account for the observed relationships between chronic disease in adults and events in early life. Further investigation should be given priority.

12.3.5 Other studies have sought to relate adult disorders to aspects of infant feeding and to the foods given. Coeliac disease is an example which is considered in para 11.1. Subjects with juvenile diabetes mellitus are more likely to have antibodies to bovine serum albumin than are non-diabetic control subjects. It is possible that as infants these children, already genetically susceptible to diabetes, become allergic to bovine serum albumin in infant formula or cow's milk. The resulting immunoglobulin may then attack protein fragments in the pancreatic beta cells because they bear a resemblance to bovine albumin[228]. The risk factor here appears to be a specific food rather than the infant's nutritional status. The relationships between when and what foods were given during weaning and the development of ulcerative colitis or Crohn's disease have been examined with varying results[229]. Some case controlled studies suggest that breastfeeding may be protective against these disorders but other studies have not confirmed these observations although the relationships have not been ruled out. A particular difficulty has been the unreliability of memory about infant feeding practices several years before. Further research should be done to clarify the relationships between weaning practices and the development of gastro-intestinal disorders in later life.

13.   Weaning and dental health

The Working Group recommends that

●   weaning foods should usually be free of, or low in, non-milk extrinsic sugars including sugars derived from fruit juices and fruit concentrates. The range of commercial foods meeting these criteria should be increased. Foods and drinks which predispose to caries should be limited to main meal times (para 13.2.2). The sugars content of all weaning foods and drinks should be shown on food labels (para 10.3.3);

●   methods should be developed to foster professional and public awareness of the importance of the weaning diet to dental health and to promote good practices especially in groups at risk of dental disease (para 13.2.2);

●   water supplies should be fluoridated to the optimum of one part per million. For infants and young children in areas that are not fluoridated, fluoride supplements may be advised where there is a particular risk of caries (para 13.4.1).

13.1   Introduction

13.1.1   Caries is the most important dental problem in young children. Despite a reported decline in caries there is evidence of a halt in this trend, particularly in younger children, a substantial proportion of whom are still affected[230,231,232]. Caries is more likely in children from lower social classes, from single parent families, families with no-one in paid employment and children of Asian ethnic origin, especially Muslims and those whose parents speak little or no English[233,230,234,235]. In inner city areas in London between 24 and 28 per cent of 3 year old children had caries[230,236]. In Bishop Stortford, where a greater proportion of children were from higher social classes, 14 per cent had caries[235].

13.1.2   Dental caries occurs when bacteria in the plaque on tooth surfaces form acid as a by-product of their metabolism of dietary carbohydrate, principally sugars. Although factors in saliva can neutralise acid, plaque may act as a barrier to diffusion so that the acid is retained, and there is demineralisation of the underlying tooth surface. The initiation and progression of caries are affected by many factors, including the type of bacteria present, the nature of dietary intake, the resistance of the host, salivary factors, and the presence and concentration of fluoride at the tooth surface[237,238]. In developed countries, where severe malnutrition is rare, the pre-eruptive effect of diet is thought to be small. Diet exerts its effects primarily through local action on the erupted tooth[239].

13.1.3   Caries although often slow to progress, may destroy the tooth within months of eruption. Rampant (or nursing bottle) caries has been associated with the prolonged use of sweetened drinks in bottles or reservoir feeders, given at bed time or nap time[240,241,242], or with "comforting" the baby with a dummy dipped in sugary material such as honey. Young children with caries often receive little treatment[243]. Once caries has become severe and especially if it has progressed to abscess formation, multiple extractions under general anaesthesia may be necessary. In a large multi-centre study in London, children under the age of 5 years made up almost one third of those receiving general anaesthesia for dental extractions[244].

13.2 Diet and dental caries

13.2.1 Caries experience has been related both to the amount and to the frequency of consumption of non-milk extrinsic (NME) sugars (para 5.5) in the diet. Sucrose is the most cariogenic sugar but glucose, fructose and maltose are only marginally less so. Between meal snacks and drinks containing NME sugars are particularly likely to cause caries. The milk sugar, lactose, and intrinsic sugars in whole fresh fruit, and in starchy foods are negligible causes of dental caries. Good weaning practices contribute to maintaining dental health. Bottle feeding should begin to be discouraged after the age of one year (para 3.6) and this is particularly important for young children who regularly consume high sugars drinks or foods such as soya infant formula (para 9.6). It is unclear whether babies who are given sweet foods and drinks retain a particular liking for sweet tastes (para 3.4). A correlation has been shown between the use of sweetened drinks and dummies as "comforters" in infancy and the consumption of sugar-containing snacks in the same cohort in later years[245].

13.2.2 Infants should be weaned on to foods and drinks free as far as possible of NME sugars. Parents are increasingly aware that they need not add sugars, or only minimal amounts where essential for palatability, to home prepared foods. Snacks should be chosen to be free of NME sugars as far as possible. Labelling of the sugars content of manufactured foods and drinks has proved difficult and confusing to the consumer[246,247] (para 10.3). Although commercial foods are increasingly presented as "free of added sugars", sugars may be incorporated, for instance, as concentrated fruit juices and these may be equally cariogenic. Manufacturers have expressed a commitment to reduce the amount of added sugars and there has been consumer pressure to develop low sugar and sugar-free products[248]. Parents who want to give manufactured foods which are free of animal products or which contain halal or Kosher ingredient may find it difficult not to rely on desserts and puddings, most of which are high in sugars. Manufacturers should be encouraged to develop a wider choice of all types of baby foods and drinks which are free of NME sugars. Methods should be developed to foster professional and public awareness of the importance of the weaning diet to dental health and to promote good practices especially in groups at risk of dental disease (para 14.1).

13.3 Sugars in medicines

13.3.1 Children who have been given medicines sweetened with NME sugars have higher levels of caries[249,250]. Sweetened medicines may particularly be used for infants and very young children and may be given at night when resistance to caries is low because of reduced salivary flow. Sugar free formulations of several proprietary paediatric medicines are now available but few generic types are sugars free and the move to change has been slow. Children who require medicines are frequently those for whom dental disease and its treatment carry the greatest potential risks and for whom effective prevention of dental disease should be a priority. The trend to eliminate unnecessary sugars from all medicines should continue and, as far as possible, all paediatric medicines should be sugars free.

13.4 Fluoride and the prevention of dental caries

13.4.1 Risk of dental caries may be reduced by the presence of fluoride at the enamel surface. The mode of action of fluoride is not fully understood but a number of mechanisms have been identified and benefits occur with both systemic and topical use. Adjustment of fluoride levels in drinking water supplies to a level of 1 part per million in this country is the most effective and efficient method of preventing caries[251] and this measure confers benefit throughout life. However, most drinking water supplies do not achieve this level. Supplements may be advised if there is individual risk of caries but there are difficulties in compliance in this long term measure or, on the other hand, fluoride intakes may become excessive. Fluoride may also be ingested from foods and drinks, and from toothpastes. There is a risk of enamel opacities if fluoride intakes are high. In a recent study relating to infant foods and drinks in the UK, analysis of 113 items showed a wide range in fluoride content although none contained sufficient on its own to be likely to contribute to opacities when used in the normal way[252].

13.4.2 Once teeth have erupted they may be cleaned gently with a small toothbrush; to start no paste is needed. The use of fluoride toothpaste is an important means of preventing caries although ingestion of fluoride toothpaste by children may have the potential to contribute to enamel opacities[253,254]. Some toothpaste formulations for young children contain lower concentrations of fluoride. Parents should brush children's teeth for them up to the age of 6 to 7 years and be aware that no more than a pea-sized amount of paste should be used.

14. Health care support and education about weaning

The Working Group recommends that

● professional staff who advise parents about weaning should be trained and should have access to dietetic expertise (para 14.1.1);

● local nutrition policies for infants and children should be culturally acceptable to the communities concerned and should be developed through local multi-disciplinary cooperation including voluntary interests (para 14.1.1, 14.3.1);

● all parents should receive nutrition education including information about weaning and the weaning diet. Education about feeding infants and young children should extend to the general public including school-children (para 14.2.1);

● more effective strategies for public eduction should be developed and they should be based on information from research (para 14.2.3).

14.1 Health care support

14.1.1 Most parents welcome individual advice from health care professionals. They may want to discuss weaning or the nutrition of the family and they need information about child health services. Parents should understand the statutory benefits to which they may be entitled, including the Welfare Food Scheme. It is important that health professionals offer consistent and accurate information in a language and style which parents understand. The health professionals must keep informed about modern weaning practices, and continuing education for all those advising parents is essential.* As part of professional education, and in order to ensure consistency of advice, public health child nutrition policies have been developed locally[257] and paediatricians, general practitioners, health visitors, dietitians, dentists, pharmacists and health educators have contributed in their preparation. Parents should also be involved in preparing these policies, as should voluntary organisations and any other interests as appropriate locally. Nutrition policies which are based in general practice should have the support of all staff including those who are not health care professionals[100].

---

* The Nutrition Task Force (NTF) Programme of Action to implement the diet and nutrition targets in the White Paper "The Health of the Nation" recognised the importance of nutrition education for all health professionals[255]. All should be aware of current nutritional guidelines and be able to communicate relevant advice. To help those involved in the education of health professionals the NTF has developed a core nutrition curriculum which can be used to amend and update any existing nutrition components in courses or to integrate nutrition to those courses where it is lacking[256].

14.2 Education about weaning

14.2.1 *Educating parents and the public* If parents are to be confident and well informed about how to feed their baby, education about infant feeding, should begin during their school years. There should be further opportunities for education during antenatal classes and after the baby is born. The personal child health record now used in child health surveillance has advice notes about feeding infants and young children[258]. Written or video educational materials should be consistent[259] and can be used to communicate information to the infant's family, to nurseries and to playgroups. These resources can be used to educate the public at large or for schools.

14.2.2 *Education to change infant feeding practices* Some feeding practices fall short of what is known to provide the best nutrition for infants, for instance starting solids too young or giving desserts and snacks instead of encouraging a diverse diet. Where it is known that there are unsatisfactory feeding practices, change may need to be encouraged. Health professionals have an important role in dealing sensitively with complex practical and attitudinal issues. Altering public perception of how infants can best be fed is difficult. Young parents often rely on community and family support, but the ways in which they are influenced may need to be modified in constructive ways. Today's parents want to know why they are being advised to change their expectations and practices. This makes it essential that advice about good feeding practices for infants and young children rests on sound research before education for change can be effective[260]. For instance, parents acknowledge and understand the hazard of too much salt in the very early diet and the undesirability of a late start to weaning beyond the age of 6 months, and these practices, once common, have virtually disappeared.

14.2.3 It is important to evaluate the effectiveness of programmes of nutrition education because, in spite of careful preparation and training, they may still fail to influence dietary practices (para 7.4). More research is needed to develop effective strategies for public education about diet and nutrition during weaning.

14.3 Particular needs for support, advice and education

14.3.1 Some families have special needs for support and education, they may not speak English, they may be new to this country or may have particular dietary needs determined by culture and religion. Those advising parents about feeding should be aware of factors (para 11.2) which influence food choices (see Annex IV). Specially prepared written materials are sometimes available[261]. Videos, teaching charts and pictures have been found to be useful to inform Asian parents, and several have been developed by and for local communities. For instance, Bolton Health Authority has prepared a resource pack on weaning available in Hindi, Gujerati and Urdu languages, and a video on infant feeding in Bengali has been made by the Tower Hamlets Health Promotion Unit.

14.3.2　The parents of children with medical or developmental disorders often need individual assistance which may include expert paediatric dietetic advise. Young children who are allergic to major food items such as cow's milk may find difficulties in ensuring an adequate diet and there are other feeding difficulties in infancy and young childhood which need individual attention. Remedial treatment and advice for some children who are not growing or feeding well may best be offered in special centres. Here child and carers come together with professional staff over extended periods to explore how best the individual child's needs can be met.

14.3.3　The cost of a diet, for a child of any age, will depend on the foods included in it. The range of foods affordable by those on low incomes will be less than for the more affluent but it is still possible to provide nutritional weaning diets at low cost. In addition, the Welfare Food Scheme provides a specific nutritional safeguard for children in low income families (see Annex V). Parents on low incomes would benefit particularly from personal advice from professionals.

15. References

1 Department of Health and Social Security. *Present-Day Practice in Infant Feeding*. London: HMSO, 1974. Report on Health and Social Subjects: 9.

2 Department of Health and Social Security. *Present Day Practice in Infant Feeding: 1980*. London: HMSO, 1980. Report on Health and Social Subjects: 20.

3 Department of Health and Social Security. *Present Day Practice in Infant Feeding: Third report*. London: HMSO, 1988. Report on Health and Social Subjects: 32.

4 Department of Health. *Nutritional aspects of Cardiovascular Disease*. London: HMSO, 1994. Report on Health and Social Subjects: 46.

5 Department of Health and Social Security. *A Nutrition Survey of Pre-School Children 1967-1968*. London: HMS0, 1975. Report on Health and Social Subjects: 10.

6 Martin J. *Infant Feeding 1975: Attitudes and Practice in England and Wales*. London: HMSO, 1978.

7 Martin J, Monk J. *Infant Feeding 1980*. London: Office of Population Censuses and Surveys, 1982.

8 Martin J, White A. *Infant Feeding 1985*. London: HMSO, 1988.

9 White A, Freeth S, O'Brien M. *Infant Feeding 1990*. London: HMS0, 1992.

10 Mills A, Tyler H. *Food and Nutrient Intakes of British Infants Aged 6-12 months*. London: HMSO, 1992.

11 Gregory JR, Collins DL, Davies PSW, Clarke PC, Hughes JM. *National Diet and Nutrition Survey of Children aged 1½ to 4½ years*. HMSO (in preparation).

12 White A, Davies PSW. *Feasibility Study for the National Diet and Nutrition Survey of Children aged 1½ to 4½ years*. London: OPCS, 1994. New Methodology Series, NM22.

13 Stephenson RD, Allaire JH. The development of normal feeding and swallowing. *Pediatr Clin North Am* 1991;**38 (6)**:1439-53.

14 Milla PJ. Intestinal absorption and digestion of nutrients. In: Cockburn F, editor. *Fetal and Neonatal Growth*. Chichester: John Wiley, 1988:93-103.

15 Milla PJ. Aspects of fluid and electrolyte absorption in the newborn. *J Paediatr Gastroenterol Nutr* 1983;**2**:272-6.

16 Milla PJ. Regulatory gut peptides and gastrointestinal transit. *Arch Dis Child* 1978;**53**:527-31.

17 Walker AF. Absorption of antigens and haptens. In: Chandra R, editor. *Food Intolerance*. Amsterdam: Elsevier Science Publishers, 1984: 17-54.

18 Forsyth SJ, Ogston SA, Clark A, Florey C du V, Howie PW. Relation between early introduction of solid food to infants and their weight and illnesses during the first two years of life. *BMJ* 1993;**306**:1572-6.

19 Hill SM, Milla PJ. Colitis caused by food allergy in infants. *Arch Dis Child* 1990; **65**:132-140.

20 Kelly DA, Phillips AD, Elliott EJ, Dias JA, Walker-Smith JA. Rise and fall of coeliac disease 1960-85. *Arch Dis Child* 1989;**64**:1157-60.

21 Beauchamp GK, Moran M. Dietary experience and sweet taste preference in human infants. *Appetite* 1982:**3**:139-52.

22 Fomon SJ, Thomas LN, Filer LJ Jr. Acceptance of unsalted strained foods by normal infants. *J Pediatr* 1970;**76**:242-6.

23 Beauchamp GK. The Development of Taste in Infancy. In: Bond JT, editor. *Infant and Child Feeding*. Nutrition Foundation Series. London: Academic Press, 1981.

24 Sullivan SA, Birch LL. Infant dietary experience and acceptance of solid foods. *Pediatr* 1994;**93**:271-7.

25 Davis C M. Results of the self-selection of diets by young children. *Can Med Assoc J* 1939:257-61.

26 Birch LL. The acquisition of food acceptance patterns in children. In: Boakes R, Popplewell D, Burton M, editors. *Eating habits*. Chichester, England: Wiley, 1986: 107-30.

27 Manning DJ, Coughlin RP, Poskitt EME. Candida in mouth or on dummy? *Arch Dis Child* 1985,**60**:381-2.

28 Department of Health. *Dietary Reference Values for Food Energy and Nutrients for the United Kingdom*. London: HMSO, 1991. Report on Health and Social Subjects: 41.

29 Department of Health. *Dietary Reference Values for Food Energy and Nutrients for the United Kingdom*. London: HMSO, 1994. Report on Health and Social Subjects: 41.

30 Department of Health and Social Security. *Recommended Daily Amounts of Food Energy and Nutrients for Groups of People in the United Kingdom*. London: HMSO, 1979. Report on Health and Social Subjects: 15.

31 World Health Organization. *Energy and Protein Requirements*. Report of a Joint FAO/WHO/UNU Meeting. Geneva: World Health Organization, 1985. WHO Technical Report Series No.: 724.

32 Prentice AM, Lucas A, Vasquez-Velasquez L, Davies PSW, Whitehead RG. Are current guidelines for young children a prescription for overfeeding? *Lancet* 1988;**ii**:1066-9.

33 Paul AA, Whitehead RG, Black AE. Energy intakes and growth from two months to three years in initially breast-fed children. *J Hum Nutr Diet* 1990;**3**:79-92.

34 Southgate DAT, Durnin JVGA. Calorie conversion factors: an experimental reassessment of the factors used in the calculation of the energy value of human diets. *Br J Nutr* 1970;**24**:517-35.

35 Black AE, Cole TJ, Wiles SJ, White F. Daily variation in food intake of infants from 2 to 18 months. *Hum Nutr: Appl Nutr* 1983;**37A**:448-58.

36 Department of Health and Social Security. *Artificial Feeds for the Young Infant*. London: HMSO, 1980. Report on Health and Social Subjects: 18.

37 Beaton GH, Chery A. Protein requirements of infants: reexamination of concepts and approaches. *Am J Clin Nutr* 1988;**48**:1403-12.

38 British Paediatric Association Nutrition Standing Committee. Vegetarian weaning. *Arch Dis Child* 1988;**63**:1286-92.

39 Williams CA, Qureshi B. Nutritional aspects of different dietary practices. In: Dickerson JWT, Lee HA, editors. *Nutrition in the Clinical Management of Disease*. London: Edward Arnold, 1988:422-39.

40 Walker AF. Effect of high crude fibre intake on transit time and the absorption of nutrients in South African negro school children. *Am J Clin Nutr* 1975;**28**:1161-9.

41 Acosta PB. Availability of essential amino acids and nitrogen in vegan diets. *Am J Clin Nutr* 1988;**48**:868-74.

42 Commission of the European Communities. *The Minimum Requirements for Soya-based Infant Formulae and Follow-up Milks*. Luxembourg, Office for official publications of the European Communities; 1989 Dec. Reports of the Scientific Committee for Food, Twenty-third series. No.: EUR 12536 EN.

43 Department of Health and Social Security. *The Composition of Mature Human Milk*. London: HMSO, 1977. Report on Health and Social Subjects: 12.

44 Holland B, Welch AA, Unwin ID, Buss DH, Paul AA, Southgate DAT. *McCance and Widdowson's The Composition of Foods,* 5th ed. Cambridge: Royal Society of Chemistry, 1991.

45 Commission of the European Communities. *Directive on infant formulae and follow-on formulae.* 91/321/EEC. Off J Eur Commun 1991;L175:35-49.

46 Black AE, Billewicz W, Thomson AM. The diets of preschool children in Newcastle-upon-Tyne 1968-1971. *Br J Nutr* 1976;**35**:105-13.

47 Paul AA, Black AE, Evans J, Cole TJ, Whitehead RG. Breastmilk intake and growth in infants from 2 to 10 months. *J Hum Nutr Diet* 1988;**1**:437-50.

48 McKillop FM, Durnin JVGA. The energy and nutrient intake of a random sample (305) of infants. *Hum Nutr: Appl Nutr* 1982;**36A**:405-21.

49 Löwick MRH, Brussaard JH, Hulshof KFAM, Kistemaker C, Schaafsma G, Ockhuizen T, et al. Adequacy of the diet in the Netherlands in 1987-1988 (Dutch nutrition surveillance system). *Int J Food Sci Nutr* 1994;**45 Suppl 1**:S1-S62.

50 Duggan MB, Steel G, Harbottle EL, Noble C. Iron status, energy intake, and nutritional status of healthy young Asian children. *Arch Dis Child* 1991; **66**:1386-9.

51 Berenson GS, Voors AW, Gard P, Newman WP, Tracey RE. Clinical and anatomical correlates of cardiovascular disease in children from the Bogalusa Heart Study. In: Schettler G, et al, editors. *Atherosclerosis IV*. Berlin: Springer-Verlag, 1983: 60-5.

52 American Academy of Pediatrics: Committee on Nutrition. Prudent lifestyle for children: dietary fat and cholesterol. *Pediatrics* 1986;**78**:521-5.

53 Lauer RM, Lee J, Clarke WR. Factors affecting the relationship between childhood and adult cholesterol levels: the Muscadine study. *Pediatrics* 1988;**82**:309-18.

54 Webber LS, Srinivasan SR, Wattinguey WA, Berenson GS. Tracking of serum lipids and lipoproteins from childhood to adulthood: the Bogalusa Study. *Am J Epidemiol* 1991; **133**:884-9.

55 Barker DJP. The foetal and infant origins of adult disease. *BMJ* 1990;**301**:1111.

56 Leung DL, Pennel MD, Leung M, Hall J. The effects of 2% milk intake on infant nutrition. *Nutr Res* 1982;**2**:651-60.

57 Davidson M. Chronic nonspecific diarrhoea: irritable bowel syndrome. In: Lebenthal E, editor. *Textbook on Gastroenterology and Nutrition in Infancy. 2nd ed.* New York: Raven Press, 1989: 1187-90.

58 Cohen SA, Kristy M, Hendricks RD, Mathis RK, Laramee S, Walker WA. Chronic nonspecific diarrhoea: dietary relationships. *Pediatrics* 1979;**64**:402-7.

59 Payne JA, Kirk TR, Belton NR. Does a low-fat diet impair growth in pre-school children. *Proc Nut Soc* 1991;**50**:233A.

60 Cockburn F. Neonatal brain and dietary lipids. *Arch Dis Child* 1994;**70**:F1-F2.

61 Farquharson J, Cockburn F, Patrick AW, Janneson EC, Logan RW. Infant cerebral cortex phospholipid fatty-acid composition and diet. *Lancet* 1992;**340**:810-3.

[62] Lucas A, Morley R, Coles TJ, Lister G, Leeson-Payne C. Breast milk and subsequent intelligence quotient in children born preterm. *Lancet* 1992;**340**:261-4.

[63] Uauy R, Birch E, Birch D, Peirano P. Visual and brain function measurements in studies of n-3 fatty acid requirements of infants. *J Pediatr* 1992;**120**:S168-80.

[64] Carlson SE. Long chain fatty acids and visual and cognitive development. *Eur J Clin Nutr*. In press.

[65] Lucas A, Morley R, Coles TJ, Gore SM. A randomised multicentre study of human milk versus formula and later development in preterm infants. *Arch Dis Child* 1994;**70**:F141-6.

[66] Englyst HN, Cummings JH. Improved method for measurement of dietary fibre as non-starch polysaccharides in plant foods. *J Assoc Off Anal Chem* 1988;**71**:808-14.

[67] Department of Health. *Dietary Sugars and Human Disease*. London: HMSO, 1989. Report on Health and Social Subjects: 37.

[68] Schmitz J, McNeish AS. Development of structure and function of the gastrointestinal tract: Relevance for weaning. In: Ballabriga A, Rey J, editors. *Weaning: Why, What, and When?* New York: Raven Press, 1989; 1-43.

[69] Payne JA. The effect of variation in sources of energy intake on the nutritional quality of the diet of pre-school children. *Proc Nut Soc* 1992;**51**:18A.

[70] Roberts IF, West RK, Ogilvie P, Dillon MJ. Malnutrition in infants receiving cult diets: a form of child abuse. *BMJ* 1979;**1**:296-8.

[71] Clark B, Cockburn F. Fat, fibre and the under-fives. *Nursing Times* 1988;**84**:59-64.

[72] Clark BJ, Laing SC. Infant feeding: a review of weaning. *J Hum Nutr Diet* 1990;**3**:11-8.

[73] Casey CE, Hambidge KM. Nutritional aspect of human lactation. In: Neville M, Neifert M, editors. *Lactation*. New York: Plenum Press, 1983; 199-248.

[74] Butte NF, Calloway DH. Evaluation of lactational performance of Navajo women. *Am J Clin Nutr* 1981;**34**:2210-5.

[75] Food and Agriculture Organisation. *Requirements of Vitamin A, Iron, Folate and Vitamin B12*. Report of Joint FAO/WHO Expert Consultation. Rome: Food and Agriculture Organisation, 1988. FAO Food and Nutrition Series No.:23.

[76] Department of Health. *The Fortification of Yellow Fats with Vitamins A and D*. London: HMSO, 1991. Report on Health and Social Subjects: 40.

[77] Rahmathullah L, Underwood BA, Ravilla D, Thulasiraj RC, Milton KR, Ramaswamy K et al. Reduced mortality among children in Southern India receiving a small weekly dose of vitamin A. *New Engl J Med* 1990;**323**:929-35.

[78] Bendich A. ß-carotene and the immune response. *Proc Nutr Soc* 1991;**50**:263-74.

[79] Ziegler RG. Vegetables, fruits and carotenoids and the risk of cancer. *Am J Clin Nutr* 1991;**53** **suppl**:251-9.

[80] Bates CJ, Prentice AM, Paul AA, Prentice A, Sutcliffe BA, Whitehead RG. Riboflavin status in infants born in rural Gambia, and the effect of a weaning food supplement. *Trans R Soc Trop Med Hyg* 1982;**76**:253-8.

[81] Jadhav M, Webb JKG, Vaishnava A, Baker SJ. Vitamin B_{12} deficiency in Indian infants. A clinical syndrome. *Lancet* 1962;**2**:903-7.

[82] Specker BL, Black A, Allen L, Morrow F. Vitamin B_{12}: Low milk concentrations are related to low serum concentrations in vegetarian women and to methyl-malonic aciduria in their infants. *Am J Clin Nutr* 1990;**52**:1072-6.

83 Hallberg L, Brune M, Rossander L. Effect of ascorbic acid on iron absorption from different types of meals. *Hum Nutr: Appl Nutr* 1986;**40A**:97-113.

84 Cockburn F, Belton NR, Purvis RJ, Giles MM, Brown JK, Turner TL et al. Maternal vitamin D intake and mineral metabolism in mothers and their newborn infants. *BMJ* 1980;**231**:1-10.

85 Department of Health and Social Security. *Rickets and Osteomalacia.* London: HMSO, 1980. Report on Health and Social Subjects: 19.

86 Grindulis H, Scott PH, Bolton NR, Wharton BA. Combined efficiency of iron and vitamin D in Asian toddlers. *Arch Dis Child* 1986;**61**:843-8.

87 Dunnigan MG, Glekin BM, Henderson JB, McIntosh WB, Sumner D, Sutherland GR. Prevention of rickets in Asian children: assessment of the Glasgow campaign. *BMJ* 1985;**291**:239-42.

88 James JA, Clark C, Ward PS. Screening Rastafarian children for nutritional rickets. *BMJ* 1985;**290**:899-900.

89 Markestad T, Hesse V, Siebenhuner M, Jahreis G, Aksnes L, Plenert W et al. Intermittent high dose vitamin D prophylaxis during infancy: effect on vitamin D metabolites, calcium and phosphorus. *Am J Clin Nutr* 1987;**64**:652-8.

90 Department of Health. *Ultraviolet Radiation and Skin Cancer.* London: Department of Health, 1993. PL/CMO(93)6.

91 Diplock AT, editor. *Fat soluble vitamins: their biochemistry and applications.* Lancaster PA: Technomic Publications, 1985:154-224.

92 Palozza P, Krinski NI. β-carotene and α-tocopherol are synergistic antioxidants. *Arch Biochem Biophys* 1992;**297**:184.

93 Muller DPR, Lloyd JK, Wolff OH. Vitamin E and neurological function. *Lancet* 1983;**1**:225-7.

94 McPhail AP, Bothwell TH. Fortification of the diet as a strategy for preventing iron deficiency. *Acta Paediatr Scand Suppl* 1989;**361**:114-24.

95 Ehrhardt P. Iron deficiency in young Bradford children from different ethnic groups. *BMJ* 1986;**292**:90-3.

96 Aukett MA, Parks YA, Scott PH, Wharton BA. Treatment with iron increases weight gain and psychomotor development. *Arch Dis Child* 1986;**61**:849-54.

97 Marder A, Nicoll A, Polnay L, Shulman CE. Discovering anaemia at child health clinics. *Arch Dis Child* 1990;**65**:892-4.

98 Mills AF. Surveillance for anaemia: risk factors in patterns of milk intake. *Arch Dis Child* 1990;**65**:428-31.

99 Wright CM, Reading RF, Halse PC, Watson JG. Iron deficiency in adolescents. *BMJ* 1989;**298**:1035.

100 James J, Lawson P, Male P, Oakhill A. Preventing iron deficiency in preschool children by implementing an educational and screening programme in an inner city practice. *BMJ* 1989;**299**:838-40.

101 James J, Laing G. Iron deficiency anaemia. *Curr Paediatr* 1994;**4**:33-7.

102 Stevens D. Epidemiology of hypochromic anaemia in young children. *Arch Dis Child* 1990;**66**:886-9.

103 World Health Organisation. *Nutritional Anaemias.* Geneva: WHO, 1972. WHO Technical Report Series No.: 503.

104 Walter T. Early and long-term effect of iron deficiency anaemia on child development. In: Fomon SJ, Zlotkins S, editors. *Nutritional Anaemias.* New York: Raven Press, 1992;81-92.

105 Oski FA, Honig AS. The effects of therapy on developmental scores of iron deficient infants. *J Pediatr* 1978;**92**:21-5.

106 Idjradinata P, Pollitt E. Reversal of developmental delays in iron-deficient anaemic infants treated with iron. *Lancet* 1993;**341**:1-4.

107 Lozoff B, Brittenham GM, Wolf AW, McClish DK, Kuhnert PM, Jimenez E, et al. Iron deficiency anaemia and iron therapy effects on infant developmental test performance. *Pediatrics* 1987;**79**:981-95.

108 Walter T, de Andraca I, Castillo M, Rivera F, Cobo C. Cognitive effect at 5 years of age in infants who were anaemic at 12 months : a longitudinal study. *Pediatr Res* 1990;**28**:295.

109 Lozoff B, Jimenez E, Wolf AW. Long-term developmental outcome of infants with iron deficiency. *New Engl J Med* 1991;**325**:687-94.

110 Parks YA, Wharton BA. Iron deficiency and the brain. *Acta Paediatr Scand Suppl* 1989;**361**:71-7.

111 Dallman PR. Iron deficiency in the weanling. *Acta Paediatr Scand* 1986;**323**:59-67.

112 Iyer S, Lonnerdal B. Lactoferrin, lactoferrin receptors and iron metabolism. *Eur J Clin Nutr* 1993;**47**:232-41.

113 Oski FA, Landaw SA. Inhibition of iron absorption from human milk by baby food. *Am J Dis Child* 1980;**134**:459-60.

114 Fairweather-Tait SJ. Iron in food and its availability. *Acta Paediatr Scand Suppl* 1989;**361**:12-20.

115 Walter T, Dallman PR, Pizarro MT, Velozo L, Pe_a G, Bartholmey SJ, Hertrampf E, Olivares M, Letelier A, Arredondo M. Effectiveness of iron-fortified infant cereal in prevention of iron deficiency anaemia. *Pediatrics* 1993;**91**: 976-82.

116 Layrisse M, Martinez-Torres C, Roche M. The effect of interaction of various foods on iron absorption. *Am J Clin Nutr* 1968;**21**:1175-83.

117 Pizzaro F, Yip R, Dallman PR, Olivares M, Hertrampf E, Walter T. Iron status with different infant feeding regimens: Relevance to screening and prevention of iron deficiency. *J Pediatr* 1991;**118**:687-92.

118 Oski FA. Iron deficiency in infancy and childhood. *New Engl J Med* 1993;**329**:190-3.

119 Hurrell RF, Cook JD. Strategies for iron fortification of foods. *Trends Food Sci Technol* 1990 September:56-61.

120 Woodruff CW, Wright SW, Wright RP. The role of fresh cow's milk in iron deficiency. *Am J Dis Child* 1972;**124**:26-30.

121 Fomon SJ, Ziegler EE, Nelson SE, Edwards BB. Cow milk feeding in infancy: gastrointestinal blood loss and iron nutritional status. *J Pediatr* 1981;**98**:540-5.

122 Ziegler EE, Fomon SJ, Nelson SE, Rebouche CJ, Edwards BB, Rogers RR, Lehman LJ. Cow milk feeding in infancy: Further observations on blood loss from gastrointestinal tract. *J Pediatr* 1990;**116**:11-8.

123 Sullivan PB. Cows' milk induced intestinal bleeding in infancy. *Arch Dis Child* 1993;**68**:240-5.

124 Fuchs GJ, De Wier M, Hutchinson S, Sundeen M, Schwartz S, Suskind R. Gastrointestinal blood loss in older infants: impact of cow milk versus formula. *J Pediatr Gastroenterol Nutr* 1993;**16**:4-9.

125 Fuchs GJ, Farris RP, De Wier M, Hutchinson SW, Warrier R, Doucet H, Suskind RM. Iron status and intake of older infants fed formula versus cow milk with cereal. *Am J Clin Nutr* 1993;**58**:343-8.

126 Irigoyen M, Davidson LL, Carriero D, Seaman C. Randomized, placebo-controlled trial of iron supplementation in infants with low haemoglobin levels fed iron-fortified formula. *Pediatrics* 1991;**88**:320-6.

127 Idjradinata P, Watkins WE, Pollitt E. Adverse effect of iron supplementation on weight gain of iron-replete young children. *Lancet* 1993;**343**:1252-4.

128 Hall DMP. *Health for all children: a programme for child health surveillance.* Oxford: Oxford Medical Publishers, 1989.

129 James J, Bailwood T, Lawson P, Laing G. Reversal of iron deficiency anaemia with iron in children. *Lancet* 1993;**41**:571.

130 Prentice A, Bates CJ. An appraisal of the adequacy of dietary mineral intakes in developing countries for bone growth and development in children. *Nutr Res Rev* 1993;**6**:51-69.

131 Law MR, Frost CD, Wald NJ. By how much does dietary salt reduction lower blood pressure? *BMJ* 1991;**302**:811-5.

132 Intersalt Cooperative Research Group. Intersalt: an international study of electrolyte excretion and blood-pressure. Results for 24 hour urinary sodium and potassium excretion. *BMJ* 1991;**302**:811-24.

133 American Academy of Pediatrics: Committee on Nutrition. *Pediatric Nutrition Handbook, 2nd edition.* Elk Grove Village, Illinois: American Academy of Pediatrics, 1985.

134 Walravens PA, Hambidge KM, Koepfer DM. Zinc Supplementation in infants with a nutritional pattern of failure to thrive: a double-blind, controlled study. *Pediatrics* 1989;**83**:532-8.

135 Walravens PA, Chakar A, Mokni R, Denise J, Lemonnier D. Zinc supplements in breastfed infants. *Lancet* 1992;**340**:683-5.

136 Aggett PJ, Crofton RW, Khin C, Gvozdanovic S, Gvozdanovic D. The mutual inhibitory effects of their bioavailability of inorganic zinc and iron. *Prog Clin Biol Res* 1983;**129**:117-24.

137 Sutton AM, Harvie A, Cockburn F, Farquharson J, Logan RW. Copper deficiency in the preterm infant of very low birth weight. *Arch Dis Child* 1985;**60**:644-51.

138 Salim S, Farquharson J, Arneil GC, Cockburn F, Forbes GI, Logan RW. Dietary copper intake in artificially fed infants. *Arch Dis Child* 1986;**61**:1068-75.

139 Haschke F, Ziegler EE, Edwards BB, Fomon SJ. Effect of iron fortification of infant formula on trace mineral absorption. *J Pediatr Gastroenterol Nutr* 1986;**5**:768-73.

140 Kumpulainen J. Selenium: Requirement and Supplementation. In: Beneficial and Adverse Effects of Various Types of Early Infant Nutrition. *Acta Paediatr Scand Suppl* 1989;**351**:114-7.

141 Wenlock RW, Buss DH, Moxon RE, Bunton NG. Trace nutrients 4. Iodine in British Food. *Br J Nutr* 1982; **47**:381-90.

142 Commission of the European Communities. *First Report of the Scientific Committee for Food on the Essential Requirements of Infant Formulae and Follow-up Milks Based on Cow's Milk Protein.* Luxembourg, Office for official publications of the European Communities; 1983 Apr. Reports of the Scientific Committee for Food, Fourteenth series. No.: EUR 8752.

143 World Health Organisation. *The Quality of Breast Milk.* Report on the WHO Collaborative Study on Breast-feeding. Geneva: WHO, 1985.

144 Lucas A, Ewing G, Roberts SB, Coward WA. How much energy does the breastfed infant consume and expend? *BMJ* 1985;**295**:75.

145 Prentice AM, Prentice A. Energy costs of lactation. *Annu Rev Nutr* 1988;**8**:63-79.

146 Filer LJ, Mattson FH, Foman SJ. Triglyceride configuration and fat absorption by the human infant. *Clin Nutr* 1969;**99**:293-8.

147 Howie PW, Forsyth JS, Ogston SA, Clark A, Florey C du V. Protective effect of breastfeeding against infection. *BMJ* 1990;**300**:11-6.

[148] Hayward AR. The immunology of breast milk. In: Neville MC, Neifert MR, editors. *Lactation: Physiology, Nutrition and Breast-Feeding*. New York: Plenum Press, 1983: 249-70.

[149] Aggett PJ, Haschke F, Heine W, Hernell O, Koletzko B, Launiala K, Rey J, Rubino A, Schoch G, Senterre J, Tormo R. The Content and composition of lipids in infant formulas. *Acta Paediatr Scand* 1991;**80**:887-96.

[150] Haschke F, Vanura H, Male C, Owen G, Pietschnig B, Schuster E et al. Iron nutrition and growth of breast- and formula-fed infants during the first 9 months of life. *J Pediatr Gastroenterol Nutr* 1993;**16(2)**:151-6.

[151] Tunessen WW, Oski FA. Consequences of starting whole cow milk at 6 months of age. *J Pediatr* 1987;**111**:813-6.

[152] Wharton BA. Milk for babies and children: No ordinary cow's milk before 1 year. *BMJ* 1990;**301**:774-5.

[153] American Academy of Pediatrics: Committee on Nutrition. The use of whole cow's milk in infancy. *Pediatrics* 1992;**89**:1105-9.

[154] David TJ. Dietary treatment of atopic eczema. *Arch Dis Child* 1989;**64**:1506-9.

[155] Milla PJ. The clinical use of protein hydrolysates and soya formulae. *Euro J of Clin Nutr* 1991;**45 Suppl 1**:23-8.

[156] Hertrampf E, Cayazzo M, Pizarro F, Stekel A. Bioavailability of iron in soy-based formula and its effect on iron nutriture in infancy. *Pediatrics* 1986:640-4

[157] Sheils K, Clements D. Calcium and soya milk. *BMJ* 1991;**303**:470.

[158] Commission of the European Communities. *Report of the Scientific Committee for Food on Infant Formulae Claimed to be "Hypoallergenic" or "Hypoantigenic"*. Luxembourg, Office for official publications of the European Communities; 1991 Dec. Reports of the Scientific Committee for Food, Twenty-eighth series.

[159] The European Society for Paediatric Gastroenterology and Nutrition (ESPGAN). Comment on antigen reduced infant formulae. *Acta Paediatr Scand* 1993;**82**:314-9.

[160] Chandra RK, Hamed A. Cumulative incidence of atopic disorders in high risk infants fed whey hydrolysate, soy, and conventional cow milk formulas. *Ann Allergy* 1991;**67**:129-32.

[161] Department of the Environment, Welsh Office. *The Water Supply (Water Quality) Regulations 1989*. London: HMSO, 1989. Statutory Instrument 1989 No.: 1147.

[162] Department of the Environment, Welsh Office. *The Private Water Supplies Regulations 1991*. London: HMSO, 1991. Statutory Instrument 1991 No.: 2790.

[162] Ministry of Agriculture, Fisheries and Food. *The Natural Mineral Waters Regulations 1985*. London: HMSO, 1985 Statutory Instrument 1985 No.: 71.

[164] World Health Organisation. *Guidelines for Drinking-Water Quality, 2nd ed. Volume 1. Recommendations*. Geneva: WHO, 1993.

[165] Toumba KJ, Curzon MEJ. The fluoride content of bottled waters. *Br Dent J* 1994;**176**:266-8.

[166] Grenby TH, Mistry M, Desai T. Potential dental effects of infants' fruit drinks studied in vitro. *Br J Nutr* 1990;**64**:273-83.

[167] Merhav H, Amitai Y, Palti H, Godfrey S. Tea drinking and microcytic anaemia in infants. *Am J Clin Nutr* 1985;**41**:1210-3.

[168] Morgan JB, Redfern AM, Stordy BJ. Nutritional composition (by chemical analysis) of home-prepared weaning foods for infants. *Proc Nutr Soc* 1993;**52**:384A.

[169] Codex Alimentarius Commission. *Recommended International Standards for Foods for Infants and Children.* Rome: FAO and WHO;1976, Joint FAO/WHO Food Standards Programme: Codex Alimentarius Commission No: CAC/RS 72/74-1976.

[170] Commission of the European Communities. *First Report of the Scientific Committee for Food on the Essential Requirements for Weaning Foods.* Luxembourg, Office for official publications of the European Communities; 1991. Reports of the Scientific Committee for Food Twenty-fourth series. No.: EUR 13140 EN.

[171] *Draft Commission Directive on Processed Cereal-Based Foods and Baby Foods for Infants and Young Children.* III/5886/94-EN Brussels,/U3/UNIC1/04/03/00/BM/dm.

[172] Ministry of Agriculture, Fisheries and Food. *Report on the Review of the Use of Food Additives in Foods specially prepared for Infants and Young Children.* FdAC/REP/I2. London: HMSO, 1992.

[173] Department of Health, Ministry of Agriculture Fisheries and Food. *Flavourings in Food Regulations 1992.* London: HMSO, 1992. Statutory Instrument 1992 No.: 1971.

[174] Common position (EC) No 17/94 adopted by the Council on 10 March 1994 with a view to adopting *European Parliament and Council Directive on food additives other than colours and sweeteners.* (94/C172/02) Off J Eur Commun: C172: 4-45.

[175] Health Education Authority. *Birth to 5.* London: Harper & Row, 1989.

[176] Department of Health. *Advisory Committee on the Microbiological Safety of Food.* Report on Salmonella in Eggs. London: HMSO, 1993.

[177] The European Society for Paediatric Gastroenterology and Nutrition (ESPGAN). Working Group for the Diagnostic Criteria for Food Allergy. Diagnostic Criteria for Food Allergy with Predominantly Intestinal Symptoms. *J Pediatr Gastroenterol Nutr* 1992;**14**:108-12.

[178] Kjellman N-IM. Atopic disease in seven-year-old children. *Acta Paediatr Scand* 1977;**66**:456-71.

[179] Brostoff J, Hawk LJ. Food allergy in children. *Eur J Clin Nutr* 1991;**45 Suppl 1**:11-5.

[180] Chandra RK, Puri S, Hamed A. Influence of maternal diet during lactation and use of formula feeds on development of atopic eczema in high risk infants. *BMJ* 1989;**299**:228-30.

[181] Arshad SH, Matthews S, Gant C, Hide DW. Effect of allergen avoidance on development of allergic disorders in infancy. *Lancet* 1992;**339**:1493-7.

[182] Ascher H, Krantz I, Kristiansson B. Incidence of coeliac disease in Sweden. *Arch Dis Child* 1991;**66(5)**:608-11.

[183] Goel KM, House F, Shanks RA. Infant feeding practices among immigrants in Glasgow. *BMJ* 1978;**2**:1181-3.

[184] Sahota P. *Feeding Baby: Inner City Practice.* Bradford: Horton Publishing, 1991.

[185] Williams SA, Sahota P, Fairpo CG. Infant feeding practices within white and Asian communities in inner city Leeds. *J Hum Nutr Diet* 1989;**2**:325-38.

[186] Treuherz J, Cullinan TR, Saunders DI. Determinants of infant-feeding practice in East London. *Hum Nutr: Appl Nutr* 1982;**36**:281-6.

[187] Warrington SM, Storey DM. Comparative studies on Asian and Caucasian children. 2: Nutrition, Feeding Practices and Health. *Eur J Clin Nutr* 1988;**42**: 69-80.

[188] Harris RJ, Armstrong D, Ali R, Loynes A. Nutritional survey of Bangladeshi children aged under 5 years in the London Borough of Tower Hamlets. *Arch Dis Child* 1983;**58**:428-32.

[189] Harbottle L, Duggan MB. Comparative study of the dietary characteristics of Asian toddlers with iron deficiency in Sheffield. *J Hum Nutr Diet* 1992;**5**:351-61.

[190] Williams SA, Sahota P. An enquiry into the attitudes of Muslim Asian mothers regarding infant feeding practices and dental health. *J Hum Nutr Diet* 1990;**3**:393-401.

[191] Sanders TA. Growth and development of British vegan children. *Am J Clin Nutr* 1988;**48**:822-5.

[192] Sanders TA, Ellis FR, Dickerson JW. Haematological studies on vegans. *Br J Nutr* 1978; **40(1)**:9-15.

[193] Dagnelie PC, van Staveren WA, Vergote FJVRA, Dingjan PG, van den Berg H, Hautvast JGAJ. Increased risk of vitamin B_{12} and iron deficiency in infants on macrobiotic diets. *Am J Clin Nutr* 1989;**50**:818-24.

[194] Jacobs C, Dwyer J. Vegetarian children: appropriate and inappropriate diets. *Am J Clin Nutr* 1988;**48**:S811-818.

[195] van Staveren WA, Dagnelie PC. Food consumption, growth and development of Dutch children fed on alternative diets. *Am J Clin Nutr* 1988;**48**:819-21.

[196] Dickerson JWT, Fehily A. Malnutrition in infants receiving cult diets. *BMJ* 1979;**1**:682.

[197] Friel JK, Gibson RS, Kawash GF, Watts J. Dietary Zinc Intake and Growth During Infancy. *J Pediatr Gastroeterol Nutr* 1985;**4**:746-51.

[198] Lucas A, Brooke OG, Baker BA, Bishop N, Morley R. High alkaline phosphatase activity and growth in preterm neonates. *Arch Dis Child* 1989;**64**:902-9.

[199] Lucas A, Bishop NJ, King FJ, Cole TJ. Randomised trial for preterm infants after discharge. *Arch Dis Child* 1992;**67**:324-7.

[200] Tanner JM, Whitehouse RH, Takaishi M. Standards from birth to maturity for height, weight, height velocity and weight velocity for British children in 1965. *Arch Dis Child* 1966;**41**:Part I 454-71.

[201] Tanner JM, Whitehouse RH, Takaishi M. Standards from birth to maturity for height, weight, height velocity and weight velocity for British children in 1965. *Arch Dis Child* 1966;**41**:Part II 613-35.

[202] Skuse D. Failure to thrive: Current perspectives. *Current Paediatrics* 1992;**2**:105-10.

[203] Edwards AGK, Halse PC, Parkin JM, Waterston AJR. Recognising failure to thrive in early childhood. *Arch Dis Child* 1990;**65**:1263-5.

[204] Grantham-McGregor SM, Powell CA, Walker SP, Himes JH. Nutritional supplementation, psychosocial stimulation, and mental development of stunted children: the Jamaican study. *Lancet* 1991;**338**:1-5.

[205] Marcovitch H. Failure to thrive. *BMJ* 1994;**308**:35-8.

[206] Skuse DH, Reilly S, Wolke D. Psychosocial adversity and growth during infancy. *Eur J Clin Nutr* 1994,**48**:S113-30.

[207] Poskitt EME. Failure to thrive. In: *Practical Paediatric Nutrition*. Butterworths: London; 1988:80-95.

[208] Cox AD. Maternal depression and impact on children's development. *Arch Dis Child* 1988;**63**:90-5.

[209] Douglas J. Chronic and severe eating problems in young children. *Health Visit* 1991;**64**:334-6.

[210] Fomon SJ, Haschke F, Ziegler EE, Nelson SE. Body composition of reference children from birth to age 10 years. *Am J Clin Nutr* 1982;**35**:1169-75.

[211] Rolland-Cachera MF, Cole TJ, Sempe M, Tichet J, Rossignol C, Charraud A. Body Mass Index variations. Centiles from birth to 87 years. *Eur J Clin Nutr* 1991;**45**:13-21.

212 Poskitt EME. Early diet - later obesity? *Br Nutr Bull* 1991;**16**:38-44.

213 Poskitt EME, Cole TJ. Nature, nurture and childhood overweight. *BMJ* 1978;**1**: 603-6.

214 Born to be fat? [editorial]. *The Lancet* 1992;**340**:881-2.

215 Davies PSW, Coward WA, Gregory J, White A, Mills A. Total energy expenditure and energy intake in the pre-school child: a comparison. *Br J Nutr* 1994; **72**:13-20.

216 Davies PSW, Gregory J, White A. Physical activity and body composition in pre-school children. *Int J Obesity*. In press.

217 Kuh D, Smith GD. When is mortality risk determined? Historical insights into a current debate. *The Society for the Social History of Medicine* 1993;101-23.

218 Ben-Shlomo Y, Davey Smith G. Deprivation in infancy or adult life: which is more important for mortality risk? *Lancet* 1991;**337**:530-4.

219 Tunstall-Pedoe H. Is the child father of the man? *BMJ* 1992;**304**:1312.

220 Barker DJP, Osmond C, Golding J, Kuh D, Wadsworth MEJ. Growth in utero, blood pressure in childhood and adult life, and mortality from cardiovascular disease. *BMJ* 1989;**298**:564-7.

221 Lucas A, Morley R. Does early nutrition in infants born before term programme later blood pressure? *BMJ* 1994;**309**:304-8.

222 Berenson GS, editor. *Causation of Cardiovascular Risk Factors in Children: Perspectives on Cardiovascular Risk in Early Life.* New York, NY: Raven Press; 1986:408.

223 Fall CHD, Barker DJP, Osmond C, Winter PD, Clarke PMS, Hales CN. Relation of infant feeding to adult serum cholesterol concentration and death from ischaemic heart disease. *BMJ* 1992;**304**:801-5.

224 Barker DJP, Bull AR, Osmond C, Simmonds SJ. Fetal and placenta size and risk of hypertension in adult life. *BMJ* 1990;**301**:259-62.

225 Hales CN, Barker DJP, Clark PMS, Cox LJ, Fall C, Osmond C. Fetal and infant growth and impaired glucose tolerance at age 64. *BMJ* 1991;**303**:1019-22.

226 Cook JTE, Levy JC, Page RCL, Shaw JAG, Hattersley AT, Turner RC. Association of low birth weight with β cell function in the adult first degree relatives of non-insulin dependent diabetic subjects. *BMJ* 1993;**306**:302-6.

227 Barker DJP, Meade TW, Fall CHD, Lee A, Osmond C, Phipps K, Stirling Y. Relation of fetal and infant growth to plasma fibrinogen and factor VII concentrations in adult life. *BMJ* 1992;**304**:148-52.

228 Karjalainen J, Martin JM, Knip M, Ilonen J, Robinson BH, Savilahti E, et al. A bovine albumin peptide as a possible trigger of insulin–dependent diabetes mellitus. *New Engl J Med* 1992;**327**:302-7.

229 Wharton B, Edwards E. Early diet and later disorders of the gut. *Br Nutr Found Bull* 1991; **16**:S74-91.

230 Holt RD, Joels D, Bulman J, Maddick IH. A third study of caries in preschool aged children in Camden. *Br Dent J* 1988;**165**:87-91.

231 Holt RD. Caries in the pre-school child: British trends. *J Dent* 1990;**18**:296-9.

232 Evans DJ, Dowell TB. The dental caries experience of 5-yr old children in Great Britain. *Commun Dent Health* 1991;**8**:185-94.

233 Paul PF, Bradnock G. The dental health of Asian and Caucasian four and five year old children resident in Coventry. *Community Dental Health* 1986;**3**:275-85.

234 Bedi R. Ethnic indicators of dental health for young Asian school-children resident in areas of multiple deprivation. *Br Dent J* 1989;**166**:331-4.

235 Silver DH. A comparison of 3-yr olds' caries experience in 1973, 1981 and 1989 in a Hertfordshire town, related to family behaviour and social class. *Br Dent J* 1992;**172**:191-7.

236 Cushing A, Gelbier S. The dental health of children attending day nurseries in three inner London boroughs. *J Paediatric Dent* 1988;**4**:77-83.

237 Davenport ES. Caries in the pre-school child: aetiology. *J Dent* 1990;**18**:300-3.

238 Johnson NW. Introduction: The Nature of the Caries Process and the Need for Markers of Risk. In: Johnson N, editor. *Risk Markers for Oral Diseases Vol 1*. Cambridge: Cambridge University Press, 1991: 1-12.

239 Rugg-Gunn A J. In: Murray J, editor. *The Prevention of Dental Disease*. 2nd ed. Oxford: Oxford University Press, 1989:4-114.

240 Winter GB, Hamilton MC, James PMC. Role of the comforter as an etiological factor in rampant caries of the deciduous dentition. *Arch Dis Child* 1966;**41**: 207-12.

241 Winter GB, Rule DC, Mailer GP, James PMC, Gordon PH. The prevalence of dental caries in pre-school children aged 1 to 4 years. *Br Dent J* 1971;**130**:271-7, 434-6.

242 Ripa LW. Nursing caries: a comprehensive review. *Paediatr Dent* 1988;**10**:268-82.

243 Winter GB. Caries in the pre-school child. *J Dent* 1990;**18**:325-6.

244 Holt RD, Rule DC, Davenport ES, Fung DE. The use of general anaesthesia for tooth extraction in children in London: a multi-centre study. *Br Dent J* 1992;**173**:333-9.

245 Silver DH. A longitudinal study of infant feeding practice, diet and caries related to social class in children aged 3 and 8-10 yrs. *Br Dent J* 1987;**163**:296-300.

246 Tyrrell A, Rugg-Gunn AJ. The current status of nutrition labelling in the United Kingdom. *Community Dental Health* 1990;**7**:351-7.

247 Tyrrell A, Rugg-Gunn AJ. A survey of nutrition labelling of sugar containing foods in the north of England in 1989. *Community Dental Health* 1990;**7**:359-67.

248 Durward L. *Sugar in Baby Foods*. London: The Maternity Alliance, Health Education Authority, 1988.

249 Roberts IF, Roberts GJ. Relation between medicines sweetened with sucrose and dental disease. *BMJ* 1979;**2**:14-6.

250 Hobson P. The effects of sugar based medicines on the dental health of sick children. *Br Dent J* 1984;**157**:155-6.

251 Murray JJ, Rugg-Gunn AJ, Jenkins GN. *Fluorides in Caries Prevention*. 3rd ed. London: Wright, 1991.

252 Vlachou A, Drummond BK, Curzon MEJ. Fluoride concentration of infant foods and drinks in the United Kingdom. *Caries Res* 1992;**26**:29-32.

253 Ekstrand J, Koch G, Peterson LG. Plasma fluoride concentration in pre-school children after ingestion of fluoride tablets and toothpaste. *Caries Res* 1983;**17**:379-84.

254 Dooland MB, Wylie A. Urinary fluoride levels in pre-school children in relation to the use of fluoride toothpaste. *Aust Dent J* 1988;**33**:101-3.

255 Department of Health. *Eat Well! An Action Plan from the Nutrition Task Force to achieve the Health of the Nation targets for diet and nutrition*. London: Department of Health, 1994.

256 Department of Health. *Core Curriculum for Nutrition in the Education and Training of Health Professionals*. London: Department of Health. In press.

257 Gibson L, Kallevik J. *Food Health Policies: The UK District Health Authority and Health Board. National Study: Progress Report.* London: Health Education Authority, 1990.

258 Polnay L. Parent-held child health records. *Maternal and Child Health* 1994;**19**:33-6.

259 Heath Education Authority. *New Pregnancy Book.* London: Health Education Authority, 1993.

260 James J, Brown J, Douglas M, Cox J, Stocker S. Improving the diet of under fives in a deprived inner city practice. *Health Trends* 1992;**24**:161-4.

261 Moss D, Pearson J. A parent's guide to nutrition in infancy [video cassette available in English and 3 Asian languages]. Nottingham Community Health NHS Trust Training Services: Phil Swerdlow Productions, 1994.

Annex I.   Studies of the Dietary Intakes of Children during Weaning*

1.   **Children aged 6 months to 4½ years in Britain (1967)**   In 1967, at the request of COMA, the Department of Health and Social Security studied 1,321 infants and young children in Britain who were selected to be nationally representative. Demographic information about this group as well as a 7 day weighed food intake record and anthropometric measurements were collected. Some of the children had medical and dental examination. Milk was the most important single source of nutrients in the younger subjects, although a more mixed diet of adult food was usual by 18 months. A few children drank very little milk and in general they were neither shorter nor lighter than the mean for their age group. Low mean iron intakes were recorded in all but the youngest group of children[1].

2.   **Children aged 8 to 60 months in Newcastle-upon-Tyne (1968-71)**   A study in Newcastle-upon-Tyne between 1968 and 1971 surveyed 140 children by monthly measurements of growth, and, for a proportion, 5 day weighed dietary records at 8, 20, 36, and 60 months. The average nutrient intakes met the then Recommended Daily Intakes[2] except that iron and vitamin D intakes were low. The lowest iron intakes were recorded at the 20 month dietary survey. The levels of energy intakes were higher in the children of "manual worker" families[3].

3.   **Five yearly surveys of infant feeding practices in Britain (1975-90)**   Since 1975 the Department of Health has commissioned a survey of infant feeding practices between the ages of birth to 9 months every 5 years. The first survey covered England and Wales[4]. The second and third surveys covered England, Wales and Scotland[5,6]. The fourth, carried out in 1990, was extended to Northern Ireland[7]. The surveys used postal questionnaires to collect the information. In 1990, at 8 weeks, 19 per cent of infants were eating solids, a reduction from 24 per cent in 1985, while at 3 months infants who were eating solids increased from 62 to 68 per cent. Early introduction of solids was associated strongly with social class, (higher rates occurring in social class V), with bottle feeding and with mothers who smoke. Early giving of solids was more likely in the North of England and Scotland. Cereals and rusks were the most common first foods. At 4 months commercial baby foods were most popular and only 27 per cent of mothers were offering home prepared foods. By 9 months of age the diet was very diverse; 94 per cent of the infants ate meat frequently–40 per cent every day.

4.   **Children aged 3 to 24 months in Glasgow**[8]   305 children were randomly selected from the birth registers for Glasgow to give a spread of subjects between the ages 3 to 24 months. A weighed dietary record was maintained for five consecutive days. A social and health questionnaire was completed and anthropometric measurements to assess skeletal size and body composition were recorded for the subject and for both parents where possible. Males had greater energy intakes but there were no differences in energy intakes for males and females when intakes were expressed per unit body weight. During the second

---

* This annex provides a brief account of some of the main diet and nutrition studies referred to in the text of the report. It is not a comprehensive account of all the surveys in this age group. The year(s) in brackets after the titles are the dates of fieldwork for the surveys.

year of life, fat contributed about 40 per cent of energy and protein about 14 per cent. About one quarter of energy intake at this age came from cow's milk. Significant proportions of the children at all ages has intakes of protein, of calcium and of iron below the Recommended Dietary Amounts for these nutrients as set in 1979.

5.   **Infants aged 6 to 12 months in Britain (1986)**   In 1986 the Ministry of Agriculture, Fisheries and Food commissioned a study of the diets of children during weaning. A sample of 488 infants aged 6 to 12 months were recruited from a commercial panel designed to be nationally representative of British babies up to 2 years. The data collected included how the baby had been fed since birth, a 7 day quantitative dietary diary record and demographic details. The sample was divided into a younger 6 to 8 month old group and an older group aged 9 to 12 months. At 8 weeks, 16 per cent of infants had received solid food and by 3 months the proportion was 52 per cent. Infant cereals, rusks and other manufactured infant foods were the common first weaning foods. Among infants aged 6 to 12 months, cow's milk was more popular among families from the non-manual social classes and infant formula among the manual social classes. The use of follow-on formulae was not common. Infants aged 6 to 8 months were eating a wide range of foods which included family foods such as breakfast cereals, bread and fat spreads, biscuits, cakes, potatoes, meat and vegetables for over half of the sample. By the of 9 to 12 months more than 75 per cent were consuming such family foods. Over a third of mothers altered the family recipes to meet the infant's needs, mainly by avoiding salt, spices and sugar[9].

6.   Daily nutrient intakes for the group as a whole are listed in Table A.1.   At 6 to 12 months energy intakes were close to the EARs (para 5.1)[10]. Fifty nine per cent of total fat intake was provided by milk and dairy produce and fat contributed 37 per cent of the dietary energy. The intakes of most other nutrients were adequate when compared with the DRVs except for zinc (para 8.7) and vitamin D (para 6.4). The recorded iron intakes were marginal, with a median daily iron intake of 7 mg which is 90 per cent of the RNI for this age (para 7.3). Fifteen per cent of infants recorded iron intakes which were below the LRNI. Average daily iron intakes of older infants were lower (mean 6.7 mg, median 5.8 mg) than those of younger infants (mean 9.3 mg, median 8.8 mg). Commercial baby foods were a major source of iron for most infants. In the 18 per cent of infants who were reported to consume no commercial baby foods, the mean daily iron intake was 62 per cent of the RNI[10].

7.   **Children aged 2 to 5 years in Edinburgh (1989)**   Other smaller scale studies carried out in the last ten years include a seven day weighed dietary record in 1989 of 153 children aged between 2 and 5 years from Edinburgh with anthropometric measurements. There were 207 quantitative assessments of the diets because in a proportion of the children the record was repeated after a 12 month interval. At 2 years the girls had a mean energy intake of 4370kJ (1045 kcal)/day and boys 4480kJ (1071 kcal)/day and energy intakes were higher among the older children. There was a wide range of total energy intake values but the energy intake per kilogram body weight was remarkably consistent and fell slightly with age[11]. The average intakes of some vitamins and minerals

101

in some groups of children were close to the LRNI. The mean daily intake of iron was low, 81 per cent of the RNI in boys and 74 per cent of the RNI in girls aged 2 years. By age 4 years the mean iron intakes exceeded the RNI in both sexes[12].

8.   **Survey of Asian children's feeding practices, Leeds (1983/4)**   Diet and nutrition surveys of Asian infants and young children are particularly important because of the known high rates of iron deficiency, higher rates of dental caries and because of the smaller achieved height in childhood[13]. Diets chosen for these young children may rely heavily on cow's milk which is sweetened and they are frequently meatless. Feeding practices in inner city Leeds were investigated by a questionnaire administered at interview in the homes of 184 Asian and 127 Caucasian infants aged 6 to 24 months. A lower proportion of Asian infants were breast fed, solids were generally first given at 4 to 5 months. For the Asian infants, the first foods were usually manufactured desserts and puddings, while for the Caucasian infants they were rusks. After 6 months more infants were being given cow's milk than infant formula in both Asian and Caucasian groups. Both infant formula and cow's milk drinks were often sweetened with sugar, honey, biscuits or rusks, more so when cow's milk was given before 6 months. Between 90 and 93 per cent of Asian infants used feeding bottles for at least 24 months[14].

9.   **Survey of Asian children's feeding practices, Rochdale (1982)**   In another study, 57 Asian and 59 white children from Rochdale Lancashire were studied longitudinally during the first 2 years of life[15]. Three day weighed dietary intakes and body size measurements were assessed on 5 occasions up to the second birthday, and blood was taken at 1 and 2 years. Asian diets were more cereal and dessert based. There were trends for the mean intakes of the Asian children to be lower than those of the white children for energy, protein, carotene and iron and mean blood values of haemoglobin and ferritin were lower. The Asian group had higher intakes of vitamin C and vitamin D which were related to a higher intakes of vitamin supplements and vitamin C rich syrup drinks. Calcium intakes were also higher and linked to higher milk consumption.

10.   **Survey of Asian children's feeding practices, Sheffield (1989)**   Children with mothers of Asian ethnic origin born in Bangladesh and Pakistan but also including 10 per cent born in Britain were studied in 1989 in Sheffield[16]. Four to five day weighed dietary diaries were collected from 154 healthy children aged from 4 to 40 months as well as measurements of weight and length, and blood was taken for analyses. Energy intakes were low, the mean exceeding 4180kJ (1000 kcal)/day only after the second birthday, and fat provided about 40 per cent of the energy. Low iron intakes were common and during the second year of life 24 per cent had haemoglobin concentrations below 11 g/dl (see para 3.7).

11.   **References**

[1] Department of Health and Social Security. *A Nutrition Survey of Pre-School Children. 1967-68.* London: HMSO, 1975. Report on Health and Social Subjects; 10.

[2] Department of Health and Social Security. *Recommended Intakes of Nutrients for the United Kingdom.* London: HMSO, 1969. Report on Public Health and Medical Subjects; 120.

[3] Black AE, Billewicz W, Thomson AM. The diets of preschool children in Newcastle-upon-Tyne 1968-71. *Br J Nutr* 1976; **35**: 105-13.

[4] Martin J. *Infant Feeding 1975: Attitudes and Practice in England and Wales*. London: HMSO, 1978.

[5] Martin J, Monk J. *Infant Feeding 1980*. London: Office of Population Censuses and Surveys, 1982.

[6] Martin J, White A. *Infant Feeding 1985*. London: HMSO, 1988.

[7] White A, Freeth S, O'Brien M. *Infant Feeding 1990*. London: HMSO, 1992.

[8] McKillop FM, Durnin JVGA. The energy and nutrient intake of random sample (305) of infants. *Hum Nutr: Appl Nutr* 1982;**36A**:405-21.

[9] Mills A, Tyler H. *Food and Nutrient Intakes of British Infants Aged 6-12 months*. London: HMSO, 1992.

[10] Department of Health. *Dietary Reference Values for Food Energy and Nutrients*. London: HMSO, 1991. Report on Health and Social Subjects; 41.

[11] Payne JA, Belton NR. Nutrient intake and growth in pre-school children, I. Comparison of energy intake and sources of energy with growth. *J Hum Nutr Dietet* 1992;**5**:15-26.

[12] Payne JA, Belton NR. Nutrient intake and growth in pre-school children. II. Intake of minerals and vitamins. *J Hum Nutr Dietet* 1992;**5**:27-32.

[13] Department of Health. *Third Report of the Sub-committee on Nutritional Surveillance*. London: HMSO, 1988. Report on Health and Social Subjects; 33.

[14] Williams SA, Sahota P, Fairpo CG. Infant feeding practices within white and Asian communities in inner city Leeds. *J Hum Nutr Dietet* 1989;**2**:325-38.

[15] Warrington S, Storey DM. Comparative studies on Asian and Caucasion children 2: Nutrition, feeding practices and health. *Europ J Clin Nutr* 1988;**42**:69-80.

[16] Duggan MB, Steel G, Elwys G, Harbottle L, Nobel C. Iron status, energy intake and nutritional status of healthy young Asian children. *Arch Dis Child* 1991;**66**:1386-9.

103

Table A.1 *Daily nutrient intakes for infants aged 6-12 months (N=448)*[9]

Nutrient		Mean	Median	SD	Lower 2.5%	Upper 2.5%
Energy	kcal	868	842	210	543	1402
	MJ	3.65	3.54	0.88	2.28	5.91
Protein	g	30.7	30.4	9.4	15.0	52.8
Fat	g	35.6	34.1	10.6	19.6	61.6
Starch	g	41.7	40.5	15.9	14.9	79.3
Total sugars	g	71.7	69.2	19.8	42.5	116.3
Dietary fibre	g	4.2	3.9	1.9	1.3	9.2
Sodium	mg	756	705	355	238	1478
Potassium	mg	1352	1340	376	681	2190
Calcium	mg	783	767	260	334	1433
Magnesium	mg	124	125	39	54	212
Phosphorus	mg	742	739	241	302	1294
Iron	mg	8.1	7.0	4.1	2.7	18.1
Copper	mg	0.6	0.5	0.2	0.3	1.1
Zinc	mg	4.5	4.4	1.2	2.7	7.4
Chloride	mg	1205	1125	533	438	2330
Iodine	μg	204	196	85	69	395
Manganese	mg	1.2	1.1	0.5	0.4	2.4
Retinol	μg	581	449	444	157	1707
Carotene	μg	1104	829	834	225	3140
Retinol equivalent	μg	765	670	463	282	1873
Vitamin D	μg	3.5	1.2	4.3	0.2	14.5
Vitamin E	mg	4.0	3.2	2.3	1.4	9.9
Thiamin	mg	1.1	1.0	0.4	0.5	2.0
Riboflavin	mg	1.5	1.5	0.6	0.6	2.8
Niacin	mg	5.5	4.7	2.8	1.9	12
Niacin equivalent	mg	12.5	12.1	3.5	7.2	20.9
Vitamin C	mg	100	81	80	15	318
Vitamin B6	mg	0.8	0.8	0.3	0.3	1.4
Vitamin B12	μg	3.2	3.0	1.2	1.0	6.1
Folate	μg	106	102	28	58	172
Pantothenic acid	mg	3.7	3.4	1.3	1.9	7.0
Biotin	μg	25.0	22.0	21.9	10.9	70.6
Saturated fatty acids	g	17.6	16.9	5.9	8.7	31.5
Monounsaturated fatty acids	g	10.8	10.4	3.4	5.5	18.9
Polyunsaturated fatty acids	g	3.5	3.1	1.5	1.5	7.4
Cholesterol	mg	165	155	70	55	332
Glucose	g	7.4	6.1	4.9	1.5	21.5
Fructose	g	6.5	5.4	4.6	1.0	19.2
Sucrose	g	18.5	16.6	9.7	4.3	43.3
Maltose	g	1.5	0.8	2.1	0.1	7.4
Lactose	g	35.3	32.1	16.8	8.6	77.3
Others/Dextrins	g	2.5	1.3	3.3	0.0	12.4

Niacin equivalent is the total amount of niacin consumed plus one sixtieth of the weight (in mg) of tryptophan.

Annex II. Essential composition of infant formulae and of follow-on formulae when reconstituted as instructed by the manufacturer*

Levels of nutrients refer to the product ready for use. They are quoted on an energy base as in the Directive. The levels in table 9.1 are quoted per 100 ml to facilitate comparison with the compositions of human and cow's milk which have traditionally been presented on a per volume basis.

		Infant formula per 100 kcal*	Follow-on formula per 100 kcal
Protein	g	2.25-3 (unmodified cow's milk)	2.25-4.5
	g	1.8-3 (modified cow's milk)	
Carbohydrate	g	7-14	7-14
Fat	g	3.36.5	3.3-6.5
Vitamins			
A	µg(RE)	60-180	60-180
D	µg	1-2.5	1-3
E	µg (TE)	≥0.5	≥0.5
K	µg	4	ns
Thiamin	µg	40	ns
Riboflavin	µg	60	ns
Niacin equivalent	µg	250	ns
B6	µg	35	ns
B12	µg	0.1	ns
Total folate	µg	4	ns
Pantothenic acid	µg	300	ns
Biotin	µg	1.5	ns
C	mg	8	8
Sodium	mg	20-60	ns
Potassium	mg	60-145	ns
Chloride	mg	50-125	ns
Calcium	mg	>50	ns
Phosphorus	mg	25-90	ns
Magnesium	mg	5-15	ns
Iron	mg	0.5-1.5**	1.2
Copper	µg	20-80	ns
Zinc	mg	0.5-1.5**	≥0.5***
Iodine	µg	>5	≥5

ns = not specifed   RE = retinal equivalent   TE = tocopherol equivalent

* Commission of the European Communities Directive on infant formulae and follow-on formulae, 91/321/EEC. *Off J Euro Comm* 1991; L 175/35

* The Directive also gives values per 100 kJ

** Infant formulae manufactured from soya proteins alone or in a mixture with cow's milk proteins have the same requirements as above except for iron and zinc which are: iron (mg) 1-2, zinc (mg) 0.75-2.4

*** Follow-on formulae containing soya protein isolates or mixed with cow's milk: zinc (mg) ≥0.75

Annex III.   The Diet During Weaning

1.   A healthy diet at any age is most easily achieved if it includes a wide diversity of foods. If the range of foods in a person's diet is great, chance alone will determine that all the nutrients needed are likely to be obtained. However, to give reassurance that all types of foods are being included, and to make the choosing of a healthy diet easier, foods have traditionally been allocated to different food groups.

2.   The group to which a food is allocated may reflect the source of the food such as "Dairy products" or alternatively, the major nutritional contribution from the foods in the group, such as "The starchy foods". Some foods span two groups, for instance, potatoes which are starchy and a vegetable. Tofu and soya products are in the "Dairy products" because they offer a source of nutrients similar to those in dairy products and they are used in the diet as alternatives for those who do not consume milk and milk products.

3.   The group called "Occasional foods" should be of secondary significance in the diet and takes account of treats such as sweets and ice cream, of accompaniments such as salt and jam, and fruit drinks as well as other foods. None of these should constitute a major component of the diet at any age but they cannot be ignored if the full dietary intake is being considered.

4.   A weaning diet should have as one of its goals the establishment of a diet with a rich diversity of foods. The pre-school child should be enjoying a broad diet which contains items from all four prime food groups. At birth, milk provides a completely satisfying diet for a healthy baby and no other foods or drinks are needed. At weaning, a diet of milk is no longer enough for the growing baby and other foods need to be included in the diet. It is important to achieve this major change in dietary practices safely and effectively with the minimum of stress for the baby and the parents. Using the food groups as illustrated in tables A and B may be helpful in achieving these aims.

TABLE A: FOODS GROUPED TO ASSIST IN CHOOSING A NUTRITIONALLY ADEQUATE DIET

	EXAMPLES	MAJOR NUTRIENTS
DAIRY PRODUCTS & SUBSTITUTES	Breast milk, infant formula, cow's milk, lassi, yoghurt*, fromage frais*, cottage cheese, hard cheese. Infant soya formula, tofu.	Energy (calories) and fat. Protein, calcium, vitamin A, B vitamins, zinc. Iron and vitamin D in breast and formula milks.
THE STARCHY FOODS	Bread, rolls, pitta bread, chapatti, breakfast cereals, baby cereal, plain and savoury biscuits, noodles, spaghetti & other pasta, semolina, rice, oats, millet, potato, yam, plantain.	Energy (calories). Protein, thiamin, niacin, folic acid, vitamin B6, biotin, zinc. Calcium, iron *(fortified cereal & bread)*, Non-starch polysaccharide *(fibre)*.
VEGETABLES & FRUITS	Leafy and green vegetables *(cabbage, green beans, peas, broccoli, leeks)*. Root vegetables *(carrots, onion, turnip)*. Salad vegetables *(tomato, cucumber)*, mushrooms, sweetcorn, marrow. Fruit *(apple, banana, peach, orange, melon)*, fruit juices.	Vitamins A and C and folate. Non-starch polysaccharide *(fibre)*.
MEAT & MEAT ALTERNATIVES	Lean lamb, beef, pork, chicken, turkey, fish, fish fingers, egg, liver, kidney, sausages, burgers. Lentils, dhal, peas, beans, baked beans, gram.	Energy (calories) and fat, protein, iron, zinc, B vitamins *(B12 animal foods only)*.
OCCASIONAL FOODS	Cakes, sweet biscuits, sweetened squash, sweetened desserts & milk drinks, ice cream, cream, sugar, jam, honey etc, crisps, savoury snacks, fried & fatty foods.	**NONE OF THESE FOODS ARE NECESSARY IN THE DIET** They may contain a lot of fat, energy, sugar, or salt. Try not to use foods from this group every day.

* These products should preferably be unsweetened varieties.

TABLE B: A GUIDE TO FOODS DURING WEANING

	4-6 MONTHS	6-9 MONTHS
MILK **DAIRY PRODUCTS & SUBSTITUTES**	**MINIMUM 600 ml BREAST OR INFANT FORMULA DAILY** Cow's milk products can be used in weaning after 4 months *(eg yoghurt, custard, cheese sauce).*	**500-600 ml BREAST MILK, INFANT FORMULA OR FOLLOW-ON FORMULA DAILY** Also use any milk** to mix solids. Hard cheese *(eg Cheddar)* can be cubed or grated & used as 'finger food'.
THE STARCHY FOODS	**INTRODUCE AFTER 4 MONTHS** Mix smooth cereal with milk; use low-fibre cereals *(eg rice based).* Mash or puree starchy vegetables.	**2-3 SERVINGS DAILY** Start to introduce some wholemeal bread & cereals. Foods can be a more solid 'lumpier' texture. Begin to give 'finger foods' *(eg toast).*
VEGETABLES & FRUITS	**INTRODUCE AFTER 4 MONTHS** Use soft-cooked vegetables & fruit as a smooth puree.	**2 SERVINGS DAILY** Raw soft fruit & vegetables (eg *banana, melon, tomato*) may be used as 'finger foods'. Cooked vegetables & fruit can be a coarser, mashed texture.
MEAT & MEAT ALTERNATIVES	**INTRODUCE AFTER 4 MONTHS** Use soft-cooked meat/pulses. Add no salt or sugar or minimum quantities to food during or after cooking.	**1 SERVING DAILY** Soft-cooked minced or pureed meat/fish pulses. Chopped hard-cooked egg can be used as a 'finger food'.
OCCASIONAL FOODS	Choose low-sugar desserts; avoid high salt foods.	Encourage savoury foods rather than sweet ones. Fruit juices are not necessary– try to restrict to meal times or alternatively offer water/milk.

** Includes breast milk, infant formula, follow-on formula and whole cow's milk

A GUIDE TO FOODS DURING WEANING

9-12 MONTHS	AFTER 1 YEAR	EXTRA INFORMATION
500-600 ml BREAST MILK OR INFANT MILKS DAILY Also use any milk** to mix solids.	**MINIMUM 350 ml MILK DAILY OR 2 SERVINGS DAIRY PRODUCT** *(eg yoghurt, cheese sauce)* Whole milk can be used as a drink & soft cheeses included after 1 year. Lower fat milks can be used in cooking, but not as main drink.	If milk drinks are rejected, use alternatives (eg *cheese*) & give water to drink. Discourage large volumes of milk after 1 year (ie more than 600 ml) as it will stop appetite for other foods. Discourage feeding from a bottle after 1 year.
3-4 SERVINGS DAILY Encourage wholemeal products; discourage foods with added sugar (*biscuits, cakes etc*). Starchy foods can be of normal adult texture.	**MINIMUM OF 4 SERVINGS DAILY** At least one serving at each mealtime. Discourage high fat foods (*crisps, savoury snacks & pastry*).	Most baby & breakfast cereals are fortified with iron & B vitamins. Cereals and bread derived from wholemeals are a richer source of nutrients & fibre than refined cereals.
3-4 SERVINGS DAILY Encourage lightly-cooked or raw foods. Chopped or `finger food' texture is suitable. Unsweetened orange juice with meals especially if diet is meat free.	**MINIMUM OF 4 SERVINGS DAILY** Encourage unsweetened fruit if vegetables are rejected. Food can be adult texture though some fibrous foods may be difficult (*eg celery, radish*).	Vegetables may be preferred raw (*eg grated carrot, chopped tomato*) or may need to be disguised in soups, pies and stews. To improve iron absorption, give vitamin C (*fruits & vegetables*) with every meal.
MINIMUM 1 SERVING DAILY FROM ANIMAL SOURCE OR 2 FROM VEGETABLE SOURCES In a vegetarian diet use a mixture of different vegetable and starchy foods (*macaroni cheese, dhal & rice*).	**MINIMUM 1 SERVING DAILY OR 2 FROM VEGETABLE SOURCES** Encourage low-fat meat & oily fish (*sardine, herring, mackerel*). Liver paté can be used after 1 year.	Trim fat from meat. Use little or no added fat when cooking foods which already contain fat such as meat.
May use moderate amounts of butter, margarine. Small amounts of jam (if necessary) on bread. Try to limit salty foods	Limit crisps & savoury snacks. Give bread, or fruit if hungry between meals. Do not add sugar to drink. Try to limit soft drinks to mealtimes.	Encourage a pattern of three main meals each day. Discourage frequent snacking on fatty or sugary foods.

** Includes breast milk, infant formula, follow-on formula and whole cow's milk.

Annex IV.   Types of diet often described as vegetarian

Partial vegetarian:

Avoidance of red meats.
Consumption of fish but not meat.

Lactoovovegetarian:

No meat, fish or poultry consumed.
Milk, eggs and other dairy products acceptable.

Lactovegetarian:

No animal foods except milk and milk products acceptable.

Total vegetarian:

No animal products whatsoever consumed.
If strict total vegetarianism the diet may exclude additives such as rennet, cholecalciferol, which are incorporated into manufactured non animal foods.
Vegans accept the need for dietary supplementation.

Fruitarian:

Cereals and pulses are excluded as well as animal products.
Fruits, nuts and seeds allowed but usually eaten uncooked.

Macrobiotic:

A restrictive vegetarian regimen is coupled with adherence to natural and organic foods.

Religions, cultures and sects which follow dietary restrictions

This list is a generalisation of dietary restrictions which are known from traditional practices, not all members of these communities adhere to them.

Christianity:

Seventh Day Adventists: Lactoovovegetarian.

Judaism:

Avoidance of pork, fish without fins, shellfish.
Foods prepared by special 'kosher' methods.
Regulations on foods which may or may not be eaten together.

Islam:

Avoidance of pork.
Foods are either 'haram' (unlawful) or 'hallal' (lawful) and must be prepared by 'hallal' methods.
Strict daylight abstinence from food and water during month long Ramadan is not practised by children but may impair feeding of children during this period.

Hinduism:

Variable restrictions. Some Hindus are strict lactovegetarians.
Pork (unclean) and meat of the cow (sacred) usually avoided.
Milk and ghee (clarified butter) are sacred foods and dairy products are usually an important part of the diet.

Jainism:

Usually strict lactovegetarians with frequent fasting.
May avoid 'hot' foods such as eggs, fish, tea, honey, lentils, carrots, onions, ginger and chilli.

Sikhism:

Variable, some are lactovegetarians.
Pork and beef usually avoided.
Meat, when eaten, must be killed by stunning 'jhatka'.

Buddhism:

Usually lactoovovegetarians.
May eat meat and fish if not killed specifically for eating.

Bahai:

Ultimate goal in the future is to reach a diet of fruit and grains only.
Many are vegan.
Fasting is obligatory at specific times for those aged 15 to 70 years (but not pregnant or lactating women).

Rastafarianism:

Very variable dietary practices.
Acceptable foods are 'total' (I-tal) or 'natural'.
Preserved foods are 'chemical' and are avoided.
Usually avoid meat. May eat fish.
Many follow strict vegan regimens with preference for exotic foods.
Cooking practices tend to involve lengthy boiling of vegetables and discarding cooking water leading to loss of folate and vitamin C.
May be reluctant to accept supplementation of total vegetarian diet.

Macrobiotic (ZEN):

10 dietary regimens (-3 to +7) of increasingly restrictive stages. Meat is allowed in the lowest stages. With increasing stages foods are gradually withdrawn. The final stage of the diet consists entirely of whole grains and liquids used sparingly.

Hare Krishnas:

Lactovegetarian who stress natural and unprocessed foods.

Annex V.   Welfare Food Scheme

The Welfare Food Scheme was introduced in 1940 to ensure that expectant mothers and young children were properly nourished. The Scheme was retained after the war on the advice of the then Standing Committee on Nutritional Problems and it has continued to the present day with a number of modifications.

Current Provisions

Expectant mothers and children under 5 years in families in receipt of Income Support receive the following, free of charge:

— *Welfare milk.* 7 pints or 8 half litres of liquid milk per week. Infants under one year may receive instead 900 grammes per week of a range of specified brands of infant formula. Breastfeeding mothers may elect to take their baby's entitlement of infant formula in the form of liquid milk to drink themselves.

— *Vitamin supplements.* Expectant mothers receive 2 bottles of vitamin drops or 90 tablets every 13 weeks for the duration of pregnancy. Breastfeeding mothers receive 5 bottles of drops or 225 tablets in total. Children under 5 receive 2 bottles of drops every 13 weeks. Both drops and tablets contain vitamins A, C and D.*

Parents of children aged under one year in families in receipt of Family Credit are entitled to purchase 900 grammes of infant formula per week from clinics at a reduced price.

Children aged under 5 years in the care of registered childminders and certain day care providers may receive one third of a pint of liquid milk (or, for children aged under one year, infant formula made up to one third of a pint) for each day spent in day care.

Handicapped children aged over 5 years but under the age of 16 years who are not able to attend an educational establishment by reason of their disability are entitled to 7 pints or 8 half litres of liquid milk free per week and to free vitamin supplements.

Liquid milk means whole or semi-skimmed liquid cow milk. Liquid milk is available under the Welfare Food Scheme from a wide range of shops and milk roundsmen.

---

*Department of Health Vitamin Drops contain
  — vitamin A (retinol equivalents) 200 μg
  — vitamin C 20 mg
  — vitamin D3 7 μg

Index

Printed in the United Kingdom for HMSO.
Dd.0300770, 2/95, C25, 3400, 5673, 313245.